What Others Are Saying

"This book is a must for those facing cancer and f... fear-filled disease. Judi writes from the heart—te... She highlights her course of action, not forcing he... , ..., r. ... ... ing options to conventional cancer care that are sound and do-able. Her recommendations for nutrition therapy and exercise are quite impressive and fact-based."

—JULIE FREEMAN, MA, RD, LD,
Licensed Nutritionist, Integrative Medicine

"This book is the most sincere and honest information that I have read to date involving a person's journey with cancer. The blessing and difference with this book is Judi's outcome. To date, she is cancer-free and is openly willing to share with others her process in achieving this. Her compelling story will inspire others to at least look at available options and regardless of their personal decisions know that hope, faith, and their attitudes will improve their lives."

—KAREN PHILLIPS
M.Ed., CLC (certified life coach), CFZT (certified foot zone therapist)
Co-author, *Life Choices: Navigating Difficult Paths*

"The wisdom shared throughout this book, and the open mind and compassionate heart from which it flows, benefits us all. Judi's holistic return to vibrant health inspires not only those directly dealing with cancer, but each one of us who seek a calmer, more peaceful and balanced life.

If we lovingly and genuinely manifest her statement, "When we improve our thoughts, we improve our feelings, which in turn, improves our behavior, and leads directly to improved results," and then apply the techniques Judi shares, we are guaranteed to enhance our quality of living, and the lives of those around us."

—PETER SHANKLAND
Massage Therapist, Yoga Instructor & Traveller
Co-author, *Life Choices: It's Never Too Late*

"Judi's story is direct, informational, and humorous. When you get to know Judi, you will see this is the way she is. This book will help those of you who are dealing with cancer to have hope, courage, and the knowledge to make informed choices. I used the practices she describes to take charge of my own health and defeat the cancer I experienced."

—LLOYD L. PALM,
Co-author, *Life Choices: It's Never Too Late*
Cancer Survivor

OVERCOMING CANCER
a Journey of Faith

by Judi Moreo

Notice: The information in this book is intended to help improve your over-all well-being. It is not a substitute for appropriate medical care. If you are facing a specific medical condition, be sure to discuss any lifestyle changes with your health care provider.

Author: Judi Moreo
Editor: Leslie Hoffman
Cover design and typesetting: Ambush Graphics

Library of Congress Number 2012953200
ISBN 978-0-9882307-1-2

Las Vegas, Nevada

www.cancerwakeupcall.com
www.judimoreo.com

Published in the United States of America

Contents

*This book is dedicated to
my role model, mentor, and best friend
who taught me to be strong, courageous,
and always trust in God.
Mrs. Daisy Shropshire-Roberts
I am honored and grateful that she was my Mother.*

Acknowledgements

THANK YOU TO DR. JOE HOLCOMB, WHO TAUGHT ME HOW TO BOOST MY IMMUNE system; Dr. Russell P. Gollard, for monitoring my blood fiercely; Dr. Neal Logan and Dr. Alan Long for chiropractic care; Heather Mirich for thermography breast screenings; Charlotte Foust and Cat Schelling for supporting me every step of the way and being the best friends anyone could ever have; Tammy Bosshardt, for nutritional and emotional support; Karen and Eddie Phillips, Carroll and Dee Statlander, Danny Statlander, Kathy Jones, Cynthia Jones, and Leslie Hare for their support and friendship; the Iron County, Utah Sheriff's Department for their dedication to duty and serving the community with caring and professionalism; Peter Shankland, masseur, for his knowledgeable attention to my mental and physical wellness; Aaron Gilliland, my dance teacher for making sure I got my exercise and helping me laugh through the whole experience; Ed Klein, my art teacher, who taught me how to see things differently and brought out my artistic talents; Tara Rayburn for the healthy homemade soups; Maria "Lulu" Serna, for caring for my home; the members of the Las Vegas Chapter of the National Speakers Association for giving me so much to focus on throughout the year; Leslie Hoffman, my editor, for making my product even better than I wrote it; Julia Lauer for the beautiful cover design; and the love of my life, Lloyd L. Palm, who has supported me in my continuing quest for a healthy and vibrant lifestyle. In addition, I would like to thank all of you from all over the world who called and sent prayers, cards, and emails of support.

Forward

AS A NATUROPATHIC MEDICAL DOCTOR, I SEE MANY PEOPLE WHO HAVE GROWN tired of the Managed Healthcare System that Western medicine currently uses to manage illness and disease. Judi Moreo is one of these people who found herself in the midst of a personal health crisis, with the diagnosis of Breast Cancer, where the options presented for treatment were not acceptable to her.

Judi, like so many others, realized her body was created by God, and while not perfect, our bodies have mechanisms to heal themselves. Indeed, there are multiple mechanisms that can be very powerful in the healing process. One of these mechanisms is focused on giving the body the micro and macro nutrients the body needs not just to heal but to function properly.

Many of the old time doctors would say, "in order for the body to heal, you just need to give it the nutrients it needs, increase elimination of toxins, and stimulate the body towards healing." In fact, all of my therapeutic modalities fit into one of these three categories. In Judi's case, we utilized therapeutic treatments in each. However, while many of the things we did were helpful in the process towards healing and health, there was one healing modality I couldn't provide. In fact, it was the most important modality used in Judi's reclaiming of her health. That modality was her faith in God and the belief she could be whole.

Now before I paint too rosy a picture of Judi, she was not always like Pollyanna. She definitely had her rough days and, at times, doubts about the decision she was making regarding her health. That being said, almost every time I saw Judi, despite some major stresses in her life, her attitude was positive and she was striving to see the glass half full. I personally feel this exercise of striving to keep a positive attitude no matter the stresses in our lives helps us weather the storms of our lives much easier and makes it possible for the Lord's Spirit to bless our lives more abundantly.

Don't mistake what I am saying. If we just have a positive attitude, we will be healed of all of our afflictions is NOT what I am saying at all. The truth is, I believe the Lord blesses us with trials and life's difficulties so we will turn more fully to Him. Sometimes those trials come in the way of our health as it did with Judi. Can there be any doubt this trial helped Judi grow closer to her Savior?

I have had patients who, just like Judi, exhibited their faith in God and believed they could live and yet, the illness they were battling took their lives. I don't believe these people had or showed any less faith than did Judi, and I don't pretend to have all the answers as to why one person may be taken and another person is able to live on. I do believe the Lord will not take us before we have fulfilled our mission in this life, whatever that may be. The Lord's ways and reasons are higher than my ways; therefore I do not question, but rather give thanks to the Lord for his great plan of happiness.

There are others who, like Judi, are healed and made well... cured if you would. And, in Judi's case, go on to touch the hearts of thousands of people, even hundreds of thousands by telling her story of faith. It might be said of Judi that the Lord has a great work for her to do, in telling those that will listen to her of her faith in Him. It has been an honor and a pleasure to associate with Judi Moreo.

I encourage you, as the reader of this book, to not just read it as Judi Moreo's story, but rather read it as a detective looking for the little clues and nuggets that are in it, which will help you in your journey. Our time here in this life is so short, the more truth we can gather while here, the more it will benefit us in this life, and I am sure in the next.

—DR. JOE HOLCOMB, NMD,
Cedar City, Utah

Another Perspective

I HAD SERVED AS JUDI MOREO'S EXECUTIVE ASSISTANT FOR SIX YEARS, SO I was accustomed to her extensive travel schedule. Often, when she would return home, she would visit her sister in St. George, Utah, a town about two hours away from Las Vegas. It was like a second home to her. While there, she would take care of personal things like having her hair and nails done, as well as going to the doctor and dentist. So, when she said she was going for her mammogram while up there, it was routine. When she called and said her schedule had changed and she was going to have surgery the next day to remove a lump in her breast, it didn't seem there was any call for alarm. She expressed no fear or emotion. She said there was no need to cancel the speaking engagements that were on her calendar for the following week. This would be an easy procedure, she would be home soon, and life would go on as usual. The surgery was much more extensive than expected. She stayed on in St. George for a few days to rest and recuperate.

A week later, we were on our way to a speaking engagement, when Judi's cell phone rang. It was her surgeon. As she listened to the voice on the other end of the phone, her expression never changed. I heard responses like "Oh," "I see," and "Thank you." She hung up, told me the pathology report was back and it was definitely cancer. That was it. Nothing more.

The only thing which seemed different that day was she wasn't allowed to lift anything. She had to stand by and let everyone else set up the product table. Two of her coaching clients and I were doing work and attempting to make sure she rested and took care of herself. We were a lot more concerned than she seemed to be. She was concentrating on doing her job...speaking. She was already moving past the cancer and the surgery.

I have no idea how or where she found the energy to deliver the program that day. She had 300 people hanging on every word and on their feet applauding at the end. You would never have known she was less than a week out of major surgery. No one, but me, knew she had, less than two hours before received that call confirming she had cancer.

Throughout the journey, cancer was never something she claimed. Once the official diagnosis was in, it was something she HAD — past tense. Every decision, every action was directed at restoring health, NOT curing cancer.

I know she had the inevitable questions, "Why me? How did this happen?" And I know there were normal fears…"I can't be sick. I need to work because I need to pay the bills and take care of my sister." I know, because we talked about it. But not in the beginning. She just soldiered on, doing what had to be done. She channeled her fears and frustrations into positive action.

Judi went into research mode. Every time I went to work, there was a new book, a new article downloaded from the internet, a new DVD, or CD in the computer. She had some serious decisions to make, and was learning everything she could to make informed decisions that would be right for her. She was dedicated and disciplined. Judi found out what she had to do and she did it.

I had my own ideas about what she should do. My partner has been through cancer twice. I had been the caretaker. I was also the caretaker for my father and my neighbor when they were battling their life threatening experiences. I supported them through the surgeries, chemo, and all the other medical issues that resulted from these treatments. We did what the doctors told them to do. We didn't stop to think. We just blindly followed the advice and orders of the doctors and did the best we could to maintain a somewhat normal life. Because of this, I felt I knew what Judi should do. I hoped when she came to her senses, she would do it. I also knew, whatever treatment decisions she made, I would be there for her. I was more than her executive assistant, we were friends. And friends support each other, not just in good times, but through the rough patches as well. This was the ultimate rough patch.

I learned that my feelings, my needs, my ideas about what she should be doing were irrelevant. What mattered were HER feelings, her beliefs, and what she needed for her own mental, emotional, and physical well-being. I learned a lot more during that summer. I learned what it means to be a part of a support team, not of a spouse or a family member, but of someone you call "friend."

I also learned of Judi's unwavering faith in God. Out of everyone I know, she has the most personal relationship with God that I've ever seen. I saw, first hand, what it means to pray unceasingly. And I saw the strength it gave her. I came to understand that hers is not faith, a belief in things unseen. It is true, committed belief. She speaks with God and God answers. I saw the results of her prayers — her energy, her passion for life, and her renewed health.

—REV. CHARLOTTE FOUST
Unity Church of Las Vegas
Las Vegas, Nevada

Introduction

HEARING THE DIAGNOSIS OF CANCER FOR THE FIRST TIME IS PROBABLY THE most alone moment of your life. It's the one time in your life when you are totally with yourself and your thoughts. No one else can know how you feel or what you should do. You will not understand it. Your family and friends will not understand it. The only one who will ever understand is God.

Even the strongest people become extremely vulnerable when they are first diagnosed. So much so that almost any authority figure can convince them that his or her treatment plan is the "only" treatment that will save their lives.

As helpful and supportive as friends and family may want to be, and as confident as the doctors are about what is right for you, you must make your own decision about what kind of treatment you will have because you are the one who will live with the consequences of the decision. No one should tell you what to do. You must make your treatment decisions yourself.

It takes a lot of courage and an incredible amount of faith to go against the recommendations for conventional medicine. It's easier to do what the doctor tells us than to do the research needed and have the discipline required to take our health into our own hands.

There are no guarantees. Some will have conventional treatments, some will choose alternative medicine and some will combine the two. Some will live and some die no matter what treatment choices they make.

It is your responsibility, no matter what you decide, to make sure you are doing everything you can to support your treatment. We should have been taught about nutrition in elementary school, but we weren't. Good nutrition supports a healthy immune system which helps your body do what it needs to do to heal. Doctors aren't even taught in medical school about the effects of nutrition on the immune system. Don't wait until it's too late, find out how you need to eat, exercise, rest and live to be optimally healthy. Just because you have cancer doesn't mean you can't have a good quality of life. You can manage the cancer. You can manage your health. You can be happy and live your life.

My reasons for writing this book are to make you aware you have options... lots of options...at almost every step of the process; to encourage you to take your time making your treatment decisions, to let you know that all feelings are okay and that no feeling is okay, to give you hope, and to help you realize you don't always have to do as you are told. I'm not trying to make up your mind for you or even persuade you to go one way or another with your medical treatment. I do want you to realize that the choice is yours and you have a right and responsibility to take your time, ask questions, and make the decision that is right for you.

Please read this book with an open mind. I am not a doctor, scientist, or nutritionist. I am a person like you who went through the cancer experience. It was not fun nor was it pretty. It was, however, my most important learning experience and I believe I have emerged from the other side a better person. This is my story. You will have your own story as you live through the process. Do your research, make your decisions carefully, and be disciplined as never before. Life is not easy and this experience is no exception. What I know for sure is that you can and will get through this. How you experience it is up to you!

You are more than enough,
Judi Moreo

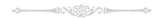

"The Power that made the body,
heals the body.

There is no other way."

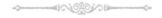

CHAPTER 1

Encountering
the Dis-ease

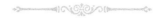

THINGS LIKE THIS DON'T HAPPEN TO ME. THIS HAPPENS TO OTHER people. People I know. People I don't know. Not me! I've never been seriously ill in my life. Oh, I've had a few sinus infections along the way, but cancer? Did she really say, "You have breast cancer?" That doesn't run in my family. We have heart attacks and strokes. We don't have breast cancer! But then, she didn't say "we." She said "You" meaning, "Me."

And so it began. From mammogram to mammogram to biopsy to ultrasound guided biopsy to surgery — both breasts. Diagnosis to surgery was so quick I didn't have time to think about what I was doing or even to feel the emotions. I heard the word "cancer." The doctor said you need to have it removed right away. I've always trusted doctors so I did what I was told.

I was to be off work the next day to celebrate my birthday, so it seemed like a good time to schedule the surgery. I arrived at the hospital at 5:00 a.m. When I awoke hours later, six nurses were singing "Happy Birthday."

The follow-up appointment with the surgeon the next week consisted of an explanation of an additional surgery which I would need to remove a sentinel lymph node — then a round of radiation treatments and chemotherapy. It was my understanding the sentinel lymph nodes are removed at the time of the mastectomy or lumpectomy. I had a partial mastectomy and a lumpectomy, but she didn't remove them then. "Why?" I asked. She said, "Because I wasn't absolutely sure you had cancer. I had to send the tissue samples to the lab for diagnosis. Now that we know, you will need to come back within the month to have one to three of your sentinel nodes removed." What did she mean, she wasn't absolutely sure I had cancer? She seemed sure when she said I had to have surgery the next day. Doubt was starting to creep in.

Even then, I listened to the surgeon and scheduled the lymph node surgery for the next month. I had always done what my doctors recommended. But now, I was starting to hear a voice inside of me telling me not to do it. As the date grew near, the voice got louder and louder. I still was not healed from the first surgery and felt I just couldn't do a second surgery at that time. I called the surgeon and asked how long I could wait before I absolutely had to have the lymph nodes removed. She said no longer than a couple of months, but waiting a month or so would not hurt. So, I postponed the surgery. She sent me to see an oncologist in the meantime. Oncologists are specialists who diagnose and treat cancer every day. If anyone has the most up-to-the-minute information on treatment options for each type and stage of cancer, it is an oncologist. This oncologist explained to me that lymph node removal is usually done at the time of the cancer surgery. It is for the evaluation of how fast the cancer is moving through the body. He seemed surprised it had not been done. He then told his assistant to schedule an appointment for me to see a radiation oncologist.

I thought the surgeon said she removed the cancer and all the edges were clean — why would there still be cancer moving through my body? If it was standard practice to remove the sentinel node when the breast surgery was done, why hadn't she done it?

> *Each precious moment of your life in which you are frozen with fear is a moment when you are not being all you can be.*
>
> —RHONDA BRITTEN

At my follow up appointment with her, the explanations still didn't add up correctly in my mind. After all, I had been led to believe the surgery would consist of a cut about an inch long where the surgeon would go in and remove a small tumor. Instead, I woke up from the surgery to find I had experienced a lumpectomy on one breast, a partial mastectomy on the other and I had large cuts along the side of each breast. On top of that, I had a staph infection in my breasts. Now, she wanted to cut me open again and was telling me it wouldn't just be one or two lymph nodes she would remove, it would be eight or ten.

She showed me a pump that looked to me like a clear hand grenade attached to a long tube which according to her, she would insert under my arm and down my side. I would have to pump toxins out of my body daily. I looked at that contraption and I couldn't think what to ask. I didn't even ask how long I would have to do this. Was it to be a week? A month? Forever? I couldn't see myself wearing that thing under my suit and going to work. What choice did I have? I didn't want to do this. I was tearful. I was absolutely positive I wouldn't do it, so I said, "You are not going to make it as a motivational speaker. There is nothing you have said that would convince me to do that." She was not at all impressed or amused by my comment and responded in a very threatening voice, "You'll be sorry you didn't." That was even more upsetting. Emotionally, everything was upside down for a couple of weeks and my immune system was growing weaker by the day.

Surely, there was another way to find out if there was any more cancer in my body, so I pestered the oncologist who said, "Yes, there is another way. We can do blood tests and a CT scan." "Well then," I said, "let's do that. Why do I want to be cut open again if you can tell from the blood tests?" Besides, I was still fighting the staph infection. What if I had let the surgeon operate again? Would the infection have spread? Would it have killed me? This made me realize that one of the most important things cancer patients should do which I had not done is to get a second opinion before allowing anyone to cut us open or treat us in any way.

The first CT scan was a nightmare. The machine broke down with me in it. I sat in a freezing cold room for an hour and a half while they repaired the machine and started over. During the second attempt, the lights in the room went very dim while I was still in the machine, so I yelled until the technician came in to tell me everyone had gone home except him and me — that's why they turned the lights out. After three hours, we finally finished the scan and I left.

The following Friday, I picked up the CT scan results and returned to my car. Reading the report, I realized it had my name and birth date at the top but the report described someone else's body. I took the report back inside and explained this was not my report. The woman who assisted me insisted that it was my report as it had my name and birth date on it and "after all, they were correct, weren't they?"

I explained to her I had never had a right breast mastectomy or bilateral breast implants as described in this report. I had never had breast implants of any kind! Instead, I had a left breast partial mastectomy and a right breast lumpectomy. She reluctantly agreed to have a supervisor call me. That call never came. I called the oncologist's office — the one who had sent me for the CT scan — to tell him what had happened, but the receptionist wouldn't put me through to him and told me, "Your problem with the imaging company is YOUR problem." I explained that it was more than MY problem as it was the oncologist who sent me there and the oncologist who would be using the incorrect information to diagnose my treatment. She finally agreed to have a supervisor call me…that call never came either. However, a few days later the oncologist called me.

I don't believe the receptionist had given him any of my messages. It seemed she had not. He simply decided to call. That made me feel better. By that time, he had received a copy of the report from the imaging company and he wanted to discuss it. Upon close examination, we realized it was exactly the same as the first report I had received except someone at the imaging company had erased the reference to the breast implants. He understood he still did not have the correct information as this obviously was not my report. He suggested we make another appointment to redo the CT scan. I refused to go back to the same imaging company as the previous experience had been a nightmare, plus they had "doctored" the report. He had a member of his staff make an appointment with a different imaging company for me to have another CT scan and a PT scan as well.

In the meantime, I went for my appointment with the radiation oncologist. Doctors should never let new patients wait in the same waiting room with long-standing patients. As I sat there, several people came in who looked very ill and had lost all of their hair. As we waited, I listened as they discussed their side effects: swelling, pain, water retention, lymphedema and neuropathy, as well as where a person could get a free wig. It was reminiscent of discussions with several of my friends who were undergoing these treatments — one had neuropathy, one had lymphedema, one died after a long and painful illness. The longer I sat there, the more sure I was this wasn't a lifestyle I would embrace. Something inside me kept insisting there had to be a better way. I gathered up all the forms I had been given, took them to the receptionist, explained I had changed my mind and walked toward the door. She quickly found the doctor, who immediately pursued me and asked that I give her the courtesy of listening to her — which I did. She, however, did not give me the same courtesy. She obviously didn't hear a word I said because when I told her I had decided not to do the radiation, she told the receptionist to make an appointment to start treatment. The receptionist gave me a card with the appointment written down. I never returned. I still needed answers. I went to doctor after doctor who told me the standard treatment for breast cancer is radiation and chemo. My heart said I didn't want "standard" treatment. I wanted treatment that was "above standard."

I continued my research, visiting clinic after clinic, spas, and raw foods facilities throughout the Southwest, Texas, and even Atlanta, Georgia. I checked out clinics and doctors in Mexico and Europe. I even saw several naturopathic doctors. One told me to go ahead and do the radiation and chemo and then he would help me regain my health. That didn't sound right to me. I prayed for guidance. I prayed I would make the right decision. I prayed for a sign or a message to help me decide what to do, but no answers came. The voice inside of me kept saying, "No" to what everyone else was telling me to do. The more they insisted I had to have chemo and radiation, the louder the voice became.

I read books and watched every movie I could find about cancer, treatment, nutrition, diet, and natural healing. I watched Louise Hay's movie, *You Can Heal Your Life* so many times I could almost quote it word for word. When I watched it, the information resonated with my heart. I felt it had answers for me. After a long month of reading, seeing doctors, watching documentaries on healing and talking with other people who had been through conventional treatments, I was more convinced than ever that an "alternative" method was best for me.

A friend who has had multiple sclerosis for 27 years and getting better every day due to a total diet change told me to check out the Cedar Natural Health Clinic in Cedar City, Utah. I looked it up on the internet and saw they offered many of the same treatments which some of the huge expensive clinics offered. I couldn't afford to stay at an out of town clinic for months either financially or time wise. I am a motivational speaker and I had bookings scheduled. This clinic said I could be an outpatient so I made an appointment. With it being only a three hour drive, it was close enough to home that I could have treatment and still manage to keep my work schedule as well as meet all of my personal responsibilities. The following week, I drove to Cedar City and met Dr. Joe Holcomb. The instant I walked into the clinic, I felt a sense of peace and a calm I had not experienced since this whole nightmare began. Dr. Holcomb is a soft spoken, kind, and gentle man. He listened intently. Then he said, "Let's see if we can get you well." What a novel idea!

The other doctors had talked to me about treatment, but no one had mentioned "getting well." I felt he was truly interested in helping me heal. After the initial examination, he put me on an intravenous drip of vitamins, minerals, and trace elements to boost my immune system. I sat for 2-1/2 hours with the tube feeding this mixture into my blood stream. Dr. Holcomb administered the drip, left the room, and came back with a book which he suggested I read.

It impressed me that he had "heard" what I had briefly shared and gave me a reference for dealing with my emotional pain. This was a doctor who did not see me as an illness. He saw me as a person. He would help me heal all of my dis-ease, not just my body.

Before I left, Dr. Holcomb gave me a large packet of vitamins, herbal tinctures, and other naturopathic medicines as well as instructions on how to use everything. He then said, "On your way out of town, I want you to stop at the chiropractor down the street and get your neck fixed. I made an appointment and he's waiting for you."

He had noticed I had a stiff neck and was suffering extreme pain. I couldn't turn my head either way and hadn't been able to do so for the past year. Again, he had made an observation of something else which was affecting my health.

The chiropractor, Dr. Neil Logan, adjusted my neck and asked why I had gone to see Dr. Holcomb. When I told him about the breast cancer, he suggested I take Vitamin D3. He was the third person that week to bring Vitamin D3 to my attention. After a short discussion regarding the benefits of Vitamin D3, Dr. Logan said, "I will work with Dr. Holcomb to get you well." I asked to use the restroom before I started the three hour drive home.

While in the restroom, I continued to pray about my decision to take the naturopathic route. Prayer was becoming a 24 hour per day activity. While praying, I looked up and saw a beautiful poster that said, "The Power that made the body heals the body. There is no other way." An incredible peace came over me. I had the answer for which I had been searching. I had my sign. I must admit I had previously thought the sign from God would possibly come in the form of a white dove, a rainbow, or something equally transcendent. I hadn't expected it to be an actual sign on a wall. But, my heart was saying, "Yes."

On the drive back from Cedar City, I stopped in St. George, Utah to see a missionary friend who lives there. When I shared this experience with her, she said, "When we feel that kind of peace, it is definitely a sign from God." She confirmed what I already knew in my heart. I had made the right decision for me. My choice of treatment may not be right for others. There were extreme lifestyle changes to be made and for some, it may be too difficult. I had to find strength enough to make those changes. I knew, with God's help, I could do it.

CHAPTER 2

Experiencing the Feelings

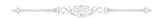

"I AM NOT AFRAID TO DIE. I'VE HAD A WONDERFUL LIFE." WHEN I said this to one oncologist, he replied that I was the first person he had heard say that. My fear was that I would live an unhealthy life — suffering side effects of cancer treatment.

When I heard the word "Cancer" in reference to me, I experienced many emotions. At first, it was disbelief. Surely, there had been a mistake. I was healthy. There was no pain. There were no lumps I could feel. All of the tests had to be wrong. After all, they had redone the tests several times and the surgeon was the only one who said I had cancer. Even she had joked after the first mammogram, "Looks like I'm not going to be able to make any money off you." I didn't think she was funny.

Once I moved from disbelief to acceptance, my first concern was what would happen to my sister if I died? Who would take care of her? I had to pay for the home I had purchased for her so she would have a place to live. Her social security check would hardly pay her living and medical expenses. She couldn't pay a house payment as well. I couldn't die. I had to get well. There was no other choice.

How you react when you are told you have cancer has an effect on your immune system. When first diagnosed, I was distressed. What should I do? How could I take time out of my life to have treatment? How could I afford treatment? If I did radiation and chemo, I'd certainly have to miss work. Then I wouldn't have an income. I didn't have much insurance and what I did have wouldn't pay for all of the treatments the doctors were recommending. It wouldn't even come close.

I was fearful of radiation and chemo. Everyone I knew who had been through it had been too sick to work, had lingering side effects, and even though some of them are still alive, the quality of their lives is substantially diminished. I didn't have the time required to go for treatment and absolutely didn't have the time or inclination to be sick. I couldn't make money if I was having chemo and radiation and was too sick to work. I had to work. I needed to make money. I had to take care of my sister and myself.

I was very frustrated and confused. I felt I had no control over my own life. It seemed no one — not doctors, not family, not friends — understood how important it was for me to make the right choice about treatment. I had more to consider than just myself. I had to find some way to get well or at least keep going at optimum efficiency as long as possible.

I started asking, "Why me? I have been a good person. I work hard. I try never to hurt others or do things that are immoral or illegal. I am a good citizen. I've really worked at becoming a quality person. I've done all I can to take care of my mom, my sisters and my brother. Now, just when I've arrived at a place in my life where I can start looking after myself and do some of what I want to do, I'm diagnosed with cancer. I know people who don't care who they hurt or what they do and they don't have cancer."

I felt trapped as though I would never be able to live the life I wanted and it would soon be over. I've always wanted to live at the ocean and felt resentful I hadn't done that. I was resentful I hadn't achieved the fame and recognition which I thought I deserved. I had written a really good book and it hadn't received the status it deserved. It wasn't a New York Times best seller despite all my efforts.

"Why me? It isn't fair. It isn't fair that I got this disease. It isn't fair I haven't achieved all I wanted to achieve in my life. It isn't fair and now it's almost over." I've always known deep down that life isn't fair, but this certainly seemed to be definite proof.

When the conventional medical doctors spoke with me, I felt like I was in enemy territory. When I tried to explain my circumstances, they told me I didn't have a choice. They insisted on treatments which would not accommodate the life responsibilities or the time restrictions I had. One doctor told me if I didn't do what she said I would be sorry. Another said that without having the chemo and radiation treatments, I would be dead within five years. Yet another said if I did have the chemo, I could extend my life for another five years. Isn't that the same five years? So, if I had the choice of living five years without chemo or living five years with it and its side effects, why would I chose to do it?

I began trying to figure out what I wanted to do with those five years. It didn't feel like panic, but it could have been. I knew for sure

I wanted to be healthy until the day I die. I wanted to be able to do the things I wanted to do whatever I decided they were. Most of all, I wanted to be the one to make those decisions...not leave it up to some doctor who doesn't really know me or anything about me. Just because doctors have diplomas on their walls doesn't mean they know what's right for me.

Because I was getting so many messages from the outside which conflicted with the messages I was getting from the inside, confusion and frustration began transitioning into anger. I wasn't mad about having the cancer. I wasn't mad at God. I was angry with everyone else telling me what to do with my life. I was also angry with doctors telling me that I only had a year and possibly a maximum of five years to live. I have never seen an expiration date stamped on anyone's forehead and I know for certain there is none stamped on mine. Where were they getting these ideas?

> *"Believe that you have the true strength to face whatever lies ahead."*
>
> —ELIZABETH GARLOUGH

I wanted to make wise decisions which led some of my family and friends to say I was in denial. I was actually only in denial for the first five minutes. I immediately did what the doctor told me and went for surgery the next day. I understood I had cancer and I had to do the best I could to make the right decisions for me in order to still handle my responsibilities. After the surgery, I started researching treatment options.

It wasn't just the doctors who didn't know me. Some of my friends obviously didn't know me either. Some told me I had to do what the doctors ordered. Others felt having radiation, chemo and conventional medicine was the only way. A few chose to say some things which I considered to be unfeeling and downright rude. One person told me that my cancer couldn't be too serious or the doctor would make me have chemo. I guess she didn't know cancer of any type is serious!

Another told me that perhaps still another of our friends could "talk some sense into me," as if I didn't have the intelligence to make decisions about my own health. My friends who had experienced chemo felt that by my doing something alternative, I was saying they had made wrong choices. They were angry with me because they believed if I made different choices and became healthy, it would make their choices wrong. They didn't understand that while it was right for them at the time, it was not right for me. Also, when they experienced cancer, many treatment options were not available that are available today.

Many people wouldn't even say the word — "cancer." Instead, they referred to it as my "condition" or my "illness." They didn't seem to understand — "I wasn't ill! I HAD cancerous tumors in my breasts. They were removed. I was angry about all of it…about the way they were treating me, about the friends who just disappeared because they couldn't cope, and about many of them trying to run my life.

Since that time, I have come to the realization that no one can truly understand what another person is going through even if they have been through similar experiences. I'm no longer angry. I have, however, made choices with regard to which of those people are still in my life and the direction those relationships have taken.

My feelings have now come full circle. I am at peace with my life and the decisions I've made. Whatever the ultimate outcome, I know my choices were driven by the voice inside, and based in solid research and scientific evidence.

Whether I live another year, or five, or twenty, I am healthy. I am in control of my life circumstances. I feel the cancer happened to me for a reason. Now, I have molded any disbelief, fears, frustrations, and anger into a platform from which I speak with passion and commitment about the process of healing the whole person... body, mind, and spirit.

The voices of conventional medicine shout at us incessantly, telling us we must do what they say. They sometimes drown out the voices of reason and choice. There is another way, and I am determined to share my story as an alternative voice in the hope it will give you the courage to listen to your body, your heart, and to that voice within you so you will make the choices which are right for you.

Most of all, I am committed to making the time I have count, not merely counting the time I have.

CHAPTER 3

Making
Treatment Decisions

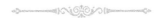

CHOOSING WHAT KIND OF CANCER TREATMENT TO UNDERGO IS A BIG decision. You must do your own research. Look at all the possible options and find out as much as you can about the results of the treatments.

I started searching for a treatment which I could fit into my schedule so I could continue working in order to pay for the treatment and my other responsibilities as well. A friend recommended Suzanne Somers' book, *Knockout: Interviews with Doctors Who Are Curing Cancer and How to Prevent Getting It in the First Place.* I read it and it gave me hope. Then another friend sent me the DVD "Natural Healing" and many of the doctors that Suzanne talked about in her book were speaking in the movie. I started contacting their clinics, but most of them were extremely expensive and/or I would have to go there for extended periods of time which would mean I couldn't continue to work. I checked out many cancer centers and hospitals… all of which talked about treatment. None would take my insurance.

With Dr. Holcomb and his staff, I felt safe. I felt we were all on the same team. I was no longer in enemy territory. These people really cared about me. We were able to communicate. You must have open communication with your medical maintenance crew. They must give you feedback and keep you informed. Most importantly for me, they need to listen as the journey progresses because our emotions and health shift and change during the course of this healing process. They have to be open to hearing what we are saying in order to effectively assist us.

> *"When we realize that we always have choices — no matter how out of control things may seem — we suddenly find that we no longer feel helpless, but empowered."*
>
> —APRIL WESTON

You must ask questions about your on-going treatment as well. Ask about its effectiveness, your cancer marker numbers, what they mean, what your goals are…both long term and short term. Ask about lifestyle changes. Ask, ask, ask. Too often information is not readily offered to you. It isn't always because the doctors don't want to tell you, it's because they are busy, they don't think you have a need to know, or they believe you already know everything you want to know. Ask any questions which come to mind. As you think of questions, write them down …even if they seem irrelevant at the time of your next appointment. Ask any questions you've had since the last time you spoke with the doctor. The answers will give you knowledge, confidence, and strength to either continue or make new decisions.

You must also make decisions about the diagnosis process. Even though many still believe that mammography is the only available source of breast cancer screening, there are other, safer choices. I have thermographic breast screenings done every three months to see if there are any changes in my body. These screenings measure the infrared heat our bodies give off and translate it into anatomical images.

The potential for cancer is detected by imaging the early stages of angiogenesis which is the formation of a direct blood supply to cancer cells. This means the potential for cancer can be detected before a tumor is large enough to be seen on a mammogram. Additionally, thermography uses no mechanical pressure or ionizing radiation, which are both factors that can contribute to the development of breast cancer.

The scientific evidence for natural means of treating cancer is not new. Researchers have been studying the effects of nutrition, exercise, stress and other factors on the growth of cancer cells as long as cancer has been known to the medical profession.

German Nobel Laureate, Otto Warburg, PhD, first discovered that cancer cells have a fundamentally different metabolism than healthy cells. His Nobel thesis in 1931 stated that malignant tumors frequently exhibit an increase in the use of glucose as a fuel. Cancer therapies that encompass regulating blood-glucose levels through diet, supplements, exercise, weight loss and stress reduction can be effective in inhibiting the growth of cancer cells.

An article by Patrick Quillin, PhD, RD, CNS published in the April 2000 Issue of *Nutrition Science News* titled "Cancer's Sweet Tooth," details the clinical research and active treatments associated with the understanding of the role of sugar, blood glucose levels and overall diet in restoring health. He emphasizes that professional guidance and self-discipline are crucial in regulating blood glucose levels via diet, supplements, medication, exercise, and stress reduction. This isn't easy, but it can certainly be done.

Wanting to be healed is not the same as having the will to "live the healing process." No one wants to be ill. Yet, given the same illness and treatment, some will live and some will not. Healing requires making the life changes required, training your mind and emotions to respond to the steps you are taking, and being totally committed to your own well-being.

Many people are willing to turn their lives over to doctors who will put chemicals into their bodies, sign waivers that detail the toxic side effects of the treatment they are about to receive, wait for hours after their scheduled appointment time for the privilege of allowing the doctor to make the decision of how to extend their lives without ever asking what the quality of those lives will be. They will faithfully commit to putting their lives in his or her hands without ever questioning the results.

There is another way. It requires making a commitment to yourself and doing whatever it takes to live a healthy, cancer free life. It means being willing to change your lifestyle, eat the right foods, exercise and rest. Do something creative every day. Pray. Love. Know that you are your first priority. Make appointments with yourself for self-care and keep those appointments. The main reason people believe holistic natural remedies don't work is because people don't make a commitment to them. It's easier to turn the responsibility for our health over to someone else than it is to do the work required when we take full responsibility for ourselves.

Once I made my choice, I was able to feel in control of my own life again and take responsibility for building my immune system. This was probably the most important decision I had ever made or would ever make in my life. I knew I had to be committed. There would be no turning back...no "should have" or "could have." I had to give this treatment my 100% participation. Thankfully, I found a doctor who supported me in doing this and an oncologist who, even though he didn't agree with my choices, agreed to monitor my blood fiercely and supported me as well.

> "We do not need to seek to become unique or rehearse to become diverse.
> God made us that way."
>
> —ANONYMOUS

Dr. Holcomb listened to me. He wanted me to heal and live my life to the fullest without putting poisons into my body. Yes, it was a long three hour drive each way to my appointments twice a week and insurance didn't cover the cost of natural medicines, but the cost of treatment was nothing compared to the cost of poor health. Actually, the cost of the natural medicine was about one-third of what the cost of radiation would have been after insurance.

If you choose conventional medical treatments, you must follow the doctor's directions. If there is daily medication, you must not skip a dose because you were too busy, you forgot, or just didn't feel like taking it that day. You must be willing to take time from your job, your family, and your other activities for doctor appointments, hospital visits, trips to the pharmacy and anything else you have to do to follow your doctor's orders. Likewise, if you choose homeopathic, natural healing, you must commit the time and energy in the same way. You must eat right, exercise, be creative, rest and care for yourself. You must be accountable to yourself. Healing, no matter what path you take, is a permanent lifestyle change. Focus your attention and energy on your health. The restoration of your health is the most important challenge you face…everything else is secondary.

Illness has a cause. If you can find the cause and correct it, then you can remedy the illness. I believe having the tumors removed, and then doing everything possible to nurture my immune system allowed my body to heal itself. To me, it seems to be a much better alternative than a program of toxic, invasive, and experimental cancer treatments.

CHAPTER 4

Dealing with the Medical Community

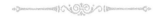

> *"Mainstream medicine would be way different if they focused on prevention even half as much as they focus on intervention..."*
>
> —ANONYMOUS

OVER 96% OF CANCER SURVIVORS start and complete some form of treatment that is grounded in conventional medicine. I had surgery to remove the tumors. My only wish is that I had taken a little more time to be certain I was more fully informed and understood each step of the process before having the surgery. I may have still elected to have it, but at the time, I wasn't emotionally ready. I was scared and the surgeon was pushing...so I did what she said and I did it quickly. Months later my breasts were still in a great deal of pain. I had no idea it would take so long to heal.

Cancer is more than cells that have mutated. Cell biology is a huge part of it, but there are lifestyle choices that are factors...attitude, nutrition, exercise, environment, relationships, and spirituality. Therefore, it takes a multi-dimensional approach to healing. It is imperative for you to approach your healing from many directions...physical, emotional, and even spiritual.

I am not suggesting you choose to eliminate conventional medicine. Certainly, if it feels right to have surgery, radiation and/or chemo, then that is what you must do. Just make sure it is your decision and not one someone else pushed you into making. I believe an integrated approach to our own wellness is required, if we are to heal.

Even with conventional medical treatment, doctors can't definitively guarantee that all patients will have the same outcome. Age, other health issues, environment, and your support system all play a role in whether or not you heal. No matter what treatment you have, the success of that treatment is as much dependent on your will to live and your willingness to do or not do whatever it takes.

Many doctors believe genetics determine whether or not we get cancer, and certainly, in some cases, that is true. In others, genetics don't appear to have anything to do with it. There was absolutely no history of breast cancer in my family. Sometimes, people who have smoked cigarettes all of their lives may very well come down with cancer that has nothing at all to do with genetics.

A Stanford University health newsletter estimated that lifestyle issues such as poor diet, lack of exercise, and unwise health habits accounted for 61% of premature deaths due to cancer. They estimated the proportional share of genetics was 29% and medical treatments themselves were listed as contributing to 10% of cancer deaths.

We all need to look at the many factors which determine the state of our health: nutrition, exercise, environment, prescribed hormones, attitude, support network, and spirituality. These key elements create the imbalance we have or the balance needed for the cancer recovery process.

Healthy cells in your body grow in predictable patterns. They are regularly replaced with other healthy cells in an orderly manner. Cancer is the mutation of genes which results in an uncontrolled, unpredictable, and irregular growth pattern of abnormal cells. They have no useful purpose and often threaten the body.

If you have an effective immune system, it will "clean up" any malfunctions of your body. However, if your immune system is down, it will not be able to protect you. You must do everything in your power to build your immune system and keep it functioning at optimum efficiency.

You must take responsibility for your own health. Your medical maintenance crew is doing everything they can to fix you, but they can't do it alone. They need your help. Most medical doctors have had very little training about diet and nutrition. One of my doctors admitted to me that he only had about four hours of study on nutrition. Therefore, it is imperative for you to study the effects on your body of what you put into your body. Your job is to do everything you possibly can to give your body the opportunity to heal.

It's also important for you to evaluate your medical maintenance crew. Who are the crew members? How many people are helping you? Are they working for you or against you? Are they giving you the information you want and need. Ask questions, questions, questions of these people. Remember, you are the one who is in charge.

You must make a commitment to getting well. You need to choose a medical maintenance crew who believes you will get well and will do everything in their power to make that happen. You need to trust they are giving you the very best of care and they know what they are doing. If you don't feel like they know what they are doing or they are not being honest with you, change teams. I changed doctors many times before I found Dr. Holcomb and my oncologist, Dr. Gollard. Part of it was because I didn't want to accept as truth the statements the others had made about how long I would live. The voice inside of my head just kept arguing. It kept saying to me, "No. No. They are wrong." Even if they had not been wrong, I preferred to continue living what seemed like a healthy life to me instead of filling my body with poisons and toxins which I believed would make me sick.

Whatever treatment you choose, be sure you have had a full explanation of your options. You want to know what the treatment is and what the side effects will be. You need to know ALL of your options. There is a vast amount of treatment information available. In fact, it can be quite overwhelming. You need to know the effectiveness of the treatments which are available. Make sure you are fully informed and understand each component of your recovery program.

Several well designed studies have clearly demonstrated that while Breast Conserving Treatment for Stage 1 and Stage 2 disease has the same success rate as mastectomy, the removal of the breast remains the predominant treatment.

There are marked regional differences, with women in larger cities more likely to receive BCT than those in rural areas. There is even a study showing double mastectomy is the fastest growing breast cancer treatment, even when cancer exists in only one breast. One woman I know had no signs of breast cancer, but because her mother and two sisters had previously had breast cancer, she opted to have both breasts removed as a preventive measure. My question is this: What doctor would perform a mastectomy on someone with no signs of cancer?

This same treatment inconsistency is seen across virtually all cancers. This is why you must do your research and demand a full explanation of all the treatment options offered you. Your treatment is your choice…be sure you are fully informed. Remember too, you do NOT have to have any treatment a doctor prescribes. Get a second opinion, and a third. Be open-minded about researching alternatives. I repeat, ask questions. Ask lots of questions. If the answers don't feel right, if you are afraid, if you have doubt, keep asking.

You know your body better than anyone else. You have been with you all of your life. You know how you feel when you've exercised, eaten a healthy meal, or accomplished something creative. Focus, commitment, and a strong faith in the Power that made your body to heal your body will bring you to a healthier life.

Become proactive in your own health. Train yourself to listen to your body. It is always speaking to you. Stay focused on your health. You will greatly improve your quality of life and you may extend your life by doing so. You must be 100% committed to your own recovery.

You must make a commitment to getting well. You must take responsibility for the state of your emotions, your physical self, and your spiritual being. Your doctor can explain treatment options, recommend what he believes is best, and treat you once you have made your decision; but you are the only one who should decide what kind of treatment is right for you. Let me remind you. You are the one who will live with the consequences of the decision.

CHAPTER 5

Building
Your Immune System

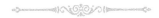

YOUR IMMUNE SYSTEM IS YOUR BODY'S MOST IMPORTANT SYSTEM. IT is your defense against millions of bacteria, parasites, viruses, microbes, and toxins which are constantly attacking your body. It works 24/7 without you even paying any attention to it. In fact, most of us hardly ever think about it unless we get sick. Yet, it is our responsibility to keep it strong so that it can combat infectious diseases and counteract toxins.

> *"The doctor of the future will no longer treat the human frame with drugs, but rather will cure and prevent disease with nutrition."*
>
> —THOMAS EDISON
>
>

Your understanding of the importance of the immune system is tantamount to your getting well. The immune system is the most powerful defense your body has. If your immune system is down, you have a much greater chance of getting cancer. Rebuilding your immune function is absolutely central to getting well and staying well.

Your job is to do all you can to reach maximum health. This is done through choices...physical, emotional, and spiritual. Use of tobacco, improper food choices, and lack of exercise all contribute to poor health. So does stress. It fills the body with adrenaline and cortisone derivatives, both inhibiting the immune system.

Your emotional response to the fact you have cancer can also be a factor in whether or not you heal. The word "cancer" creates paralyzing fear in most people, emotionally as well as physically. It is at this time when we most need to intellectually diagnose our situation, take the time to do our homework, find out what our choices are, and have the courage to take the action we believe is right for us.

Negative physiological responses negatively impact the immune system. Your lifestyle affects the activity of your immune system. If you smoke, give it up. If you eat harmful foods, give them up and make healthier choices. If you have a great deal of stress in your life, change your activities. If you have a negative attitude, fix it!

When you decide on a treatment program, be sure you believe in it. When Dr. Holcomb told me I would be having drips of vitamins, minerals, and trace elements, I knew they were healthy things and would be good for me. Certainly changing my eating habits couldn't hurt me. I was convinced this was the right thing to do. In fact, I was excited about the journey. I was sure he was the right doctor and the treatment he prescribed would make me well.

Do you truly know which foods nourish your body and which don't? I didn't. I thought I did, but I really didn't. As I learned more and more about nutrition, healthy choices became my ally. I wasn't being punished by not eating certain foods. I was being rewarded by eating foods which were good for me. Every day, I was getting stronger and feeling better.

Are you making it a habit to eat only those things which fuel your energy? Or do you stuff yourself with foods you know you shouldn't eat? Would you put trash in the gas tank of your car? If not, why would you put trash in the fuel tank of your body?

Are you aware of what vitamin and mineral supplements you need? Are you making sure you take them daily? As a cancer survivor, I now realize we must all pay attention to our nutrition if we want to be healthy and stay healthy.

> *"The food you eat can be either the safest and most powerful form of medicine or the slowest form of poison."*
>
> —ANN WIGMORE

We must think about what we are eating. There are approximately four million cancer patients in America today and numerous more throughout the world, yet hardly any are offered any nutritional advice by the medical community. We are told to "eat good food." What does that mean? I'm sure it doesn't mean to continue doing what we were doing in the past, because that obviously didn't work. So, what changes should we make? What is "good food"? Many people believe they are eating good food when, in fact, the food they are eating is not nutritional at all.

We should eat a diet that supplies the essential nutrients: fresh vegetables, fruits, and whole grains. Drink pure water. Leave off fat, salt, and sugar. Sugar feeds cancer! Did you get that? Sugar feeds cancer! Cut it out of your diet immediately! Also, cut out anything which turns to sugar in your body. That means simple carbohydrates. Eat more vegetables than fruits.

We need to stay away from packaged foods because they contain preservatives and have less nutritional value than fresh foods. Controlling our blood-glucose levels through diet, supplements, exercise and meditation is crucial to our cancer recovery programs.

I changed my eating habits – eliminating sugar, salt, all white foods, all packaged foods, red meat, dairy products, alcohol and caffeinated drinks. I eat mostly raw vegetables, fish, and some organic chicken. I have become very fond of fresh strawberries. My mantra became: *If it is boxed, bottled, canned, or packaged, I shouldn't be eating it.*

The following is the eating program I designed for myself from what my doctors recommended and what I had read in the many books I was devouring. If you decide to try it, remember all fruits and vegetables should be organic, if at all possible. If you can't obtain organic, then thoroughly wash them to be sure you have cleaned away any pesticides and herbicides.

Eating Program

VEGETABLES		FRUITS
Artichokes	Swiss Chard	Apricots
Avocados	Okra	Lemons
Arugula	Sweet potato	Limes
Broccoli	Yams	Berries (especially
Cabbage		strawberries)
Cucumber		Papaya
Peppers		Pineapple
Asparagus		Red Grapefruit
Leaf lettuce		Tomatoes
Cauliflower		Cherries
Onions		Pears
Beets		Cantaloupe
Kale		Mangos
Spinach		Watermelon
Sprouts		Apples
Squash		Bananas
Green beans		

Green vegetables that grow above ground are actually better for you than vegetables that grow underground due to the sugar content of those growing beneath the soil.

FISH, MEAT & EGGS	WHOLE GRAINS AND BREADS
Salmon (wild)	Oats
Halibut (wild)	Brown Rice
Trout (wild)	Flaxseed
Sea bass (wild)	Quinoa
Eggs (organic)	
Skinless chicken (organic)	
Turkey breast (organic)	

LEGUMES	OTHER
Black beans	Garlic
Garbanzo beans	Ginger
Kidney beans	Cinnamon
Navy beans	Cayenne
Pinto beans	Stevia
Lentils	Curry
Split peas	Turmeric
	Green Tea
	Agave

NUTS AND SEEDS	OILS
Almonds	Extra virgin olive oil
Pecans	Sesame oil
Sesame seeds	Flaxseed oil
Sunflower seeds	
Flax – must be fresh ground seeds	

Herbs

Garlic is nature's antibiotic and can inhibit viruses and help prevent cancer. It is perhaps the strongest single food you can add to your eating program to boost your immune system. Other herbs reputed to boost the immune system include turmeric, echinacea, goldenseal, astragalus, ginseng, ginkgo and gotu kola.

Water

Drink eight cups of pure water each day.

Don't tell me you don't like water. It's not about your likes and dislikes. It's about what makes your body function properly. People tell me if they drink orange juice or tea or coffee, it's the same thing as drinking water. I disagree. Try washing your clothes in any of those... then tell me it's the same.

Do Not Eat

All processed or manufactured foods should be avoided. Don't eat any foods that are bottled, canned, frozen, preserved, refined, salted, or smoked.

Dairy products create mucus. Cancer thrives in mucus. Avoid dairy products. This includes milk, cheese, ice cream, ice milk, butter, and buttermilk.

Alcohol limits the blood's ability to carry oxygen. It also places strain on the liver to remove toxins from the body.

Oils and fats should be eliminated, except for those recommended in the previous list.

Products made from flour, baking powder, baking soda, and refined white and brown sugars should not be eaten.

Beef, pork, poultry, farm fed fish or any other animal flesh products should be eliminated. They are high in protein, fats, chemicals, preservatives, hormones, salt, and are difficult to digest.

Mushrooms are fungi and contain complex proteins which are difficult to digest. Many are reputed to have immune modulating activity, but I suggest you talk with your alternative health care provider in order to know which ones do what.

Foods I Eliminated

Sugar	Liquor
Aspartame	Beer
Syrups	Wine
Hydrogenated fats	Soft drinks, regular
Lard	Soft drinks, diet
Margarine	Ice cream
Red Meat	Cookies
Pizza	Doughnuts
Bologna	Cake
Sausage	Boxed cereal
Bacon	Molasses
Smoked Ham	Wheat

Undergoing this eating program was something I had to do. I didn't have any idea how easy it would be. I made it a point not to have anything in the house that wasn't on the DO eat list. In restaurants, I looked at my DO list and picked what was on the menu that matched up to the list. It's amazing how accommodating restaurant employees can be. Before long, I had lost seventeen pounds and felt better than I had in years.

Two of my friends decided to support me in this new way of eating and to their surprise, they both lost weight. One lost 38 pounds and one lost 55 pounds in only six months. The one who lost the most is also a cancer survivor and she found by eating this way, her neuropathy greatly improved. She was also attended by the same oncologist as me. When she went in for her yearly checkup, he was surprised at her improvement and asked what she was doing. She said she had been eating the food on my eating program. He looked at her and said, "Well, there must be something to this nutrition thing."

A fact sheet published by Cornell University in June 2002 states, "While diet and lifestyle have been associated with the risk of getting breast cancer, little is known about the effect of diet and lifestyle on breast cancer survival." Understanding the consequences of diet and lifestyle on breast cancer survival is important to survivors of breast cancer who want to make choices to improve the length and quality of their lives.

As you begin to eat healthier foods and drink more water, it's amazing how your cravings for the things you think you can't live without will begin to go away. You may go through withdrawal, like you would with any addictive drug. In the long run, you'll probably find you really enjoy fresh foods, water, and the flavor of food not masked by salt, sugar or other addictive additives.

Understanding and applying better nutritional choices to your diet is the one change you must make no matter what you choose as your treatment plan. Supporting your general health while undergoing any treatment will enhance your body's ability to heal and help to minimize any side effects of drugs and radiation. Take responsibility for boosting your immune system!

CHAPTER 6

Supplementing Your Diet

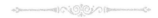

OUR BODIES NEED VITAMINS, MINERALS, AND A BALANCE OF PROTEINS and carbohydrates in order to rebuild cells and function properly. Many times, there is a deficiency involved with a lower immune system. Incorporating vitamins such as A, B, C, D3 and E, as well as minerals such as magnesium, selenium, zinc, and folic acid into our diets will help to optimize our immune response. We must also take a serious look at the role vitamins, minerals, and herbal supplements play in the management of cancer. Be sure to check with your doctor or nutritionist first, but seriously consider supplementing your diet with any missing vitamins or nutrients and be sure they are in the most bioavailable form for proper absorption and utilization.

> *"Today, more than 95% of all chronic disease is caused by food choices, toxic food ingredients, nutritional deficiencies, and lack of physical exercise."*
>
> —MIKE ADAMS

Vitamin A

Vitamin A is the defensive line of the immune system. Vitamin A keeps viruses, infections, and other germs from getting into our bodies. Vitamin A keeps mucous membranes that line the throat, nose, mouth and other parts of the body soft and moist. When these membranes are kept soft and moist, they are better able to trap germs, stopping their infiltration. Furthermore, Vitamin A helps to boost the immune system by making enzymes which look for and kill germs that manage to get inside the body.

B-Vitamins

B-vitamins are energy-boosting vitamins that also boost the immune system. Vitamins such as folate, B6 and B12 strengthen and boost the immune system. Vitamin B6 especially, has been shown in studies to boost the immune system by increasing white blood cell count in the body. The Department of Nutrition and Food Management at Oregon State University conducted a study and found when women increased their B6 intake from 1.5 milligrams to 2.1 milligrams, their white blood cell count increased by 35%.

Vitamin B6 aids other vitamins and helps the immune system with the growth of new cells. Vitamin B6 can help convert tryptophan to niacin (vitamin B3). It also helps serotonin levels, which aids sleep and blood cells, allowing the body to heal itself faster. This vitamin is vital for women as it balances hormonal changes while affecting mood and behavior.

Vitamin C

Vitamin C, also known as ascorbic acid, is a natural immune system booster. Not only does this vitamin help with the basic immune system, it may also protect against various types of cancers such as mouth, esophagus, stomach, and breast. This vitamin helps make collagen which is used by the body as a connective tissue to heal wounds and support blood vessel walls. It also acts as an anti-oxidant which neutralizes unstable molecules that can damage cell walls.

Vitamin C is not a part of the defensive line for the immune system. Rather, Vitamin C takes the offensive line against germs. Vitamin C boosts the immune system by boosting the cells responsible for killing germs in the body. Vitamin C makes interferon, a protein that helps destroy viruses in the body. It also increases the level of glutathione, which boosts the immune system. Vitamin C and other antioxidants protect your cells from toxin damage, making the cells stronger. So, remember your citrus (oranges, grapefruits, lemons, etc.) and berries (especially the darker berries.) Lemons have the added benefit of helping balance your body's acid/alkali levels. This is important because a healthy pH level supports the right bacteria. Too often, the body is more acidic than it should be, creating an environment conducive to viruses and invading bacteria. Though it may seem backwards, diets rich in acidic foods, like lemons, produce a less acidic pH, while a diet rich in breads and meats produces a more acidic pH.

Dr. Holcomb told me to drink three packets of EmergenC per day. EmergenC is a vitamin drink mix full of 24 different nutrients and 1,000 mg of Vitamin C in each packet. EmergenC also contains seven B vitamins, used to naturally enhance your overall energy without the use of caffeine. After one month, he increased my dosage to six packets of EmergenC per day. After another month, nine packets of EmergenC per day. I believe the Vitamin C was a huge factor in my rapid healing.

Vitamin D

The so-called sunshine vitamin, which can be obtained from food or manufactured by human skin exposed to the sun, plays a key role in boosting the immune system, researchers believe. In particular it triggers and arms the body's T cells, the cells in the body that seek out and destroy any invading bacteria and viruses.

Dr. Richard Besser, ABC News' Senior Health and Medical Editor, suggests that people get enough sunlight - which he says is thirty minutes of sun twice a week — generally between the hours of 10:00 a.m. and 3:00 p.m. He also said such levels of exposure won't increase the risk for cancer...people who can't get enough of the vitamin through diet and sun exposure, should consider a supplement.

Scientists at the University of Copenhagen have discovered that Vitamin D is crucial to activating our immune defenses and without sufficient intake of the vitamin, the killer cells of the immune system — T cells — will not be able to react to and fight off serious infections in the body.

For T cells to detect and kill foreign pathogens such as clumps of bacteria or viruses, the cells must first be "triggered" into action and "transform" from inactive and harmless immune cells into killer cells that are primed to seek out and destroy all traces of invaders. The researchers found that T cells rely on Vitamin D in order to activate, and they remain dormant, 'naïve' to the possibility of threat, if Vitamin D is lacking in the blood.

The medical community knows that low levels of Vitamin D are linked to certain kinds of cancers as well as to other diseases such as asthma and diabetes, but research by JoEllen Welsh, a researcher with the State University of New York at Albany, shows that Vitamin D can cause cancer cells to shrivel up and die. Welsh said Vitamin D has the same effect as a drug used for breast cancer treatment.

Vitamin D3

Vitamin D3, an essential vitamin the body needs to function properly, is the natural human form of Vitamin D made in the skin when cholesterol reacts with sunlight. Most people get their daily dose of D by being out in the sun, as ultraviolet rays trigger the creation of Vitamin D3 in the body. Maintaining the proper levels of Vitamin D3 is essential, as a deficiency has been linked to all sorts of problems from rickets and obesity to cancer. (Do not confuse D3 with D2 which may be found in small amounts in multivitamins.)

You need Vitamin D3 to properly absorb calcium. Further, it reduces inflammation and builds the immune system. Vitamin D3 is important for your overall health and well-being.

The Life Extension Foundation suggests breast cancer patients take between 4000 to 6000 IU of Vitamin D3 per day. Periodic blood tests are needed. Always consult your health care advisor and keep him or her advised of your dosage regimen.

Vitamin E

Vitamin E has also been known to boost the immune system by producing Interleukin-2, an immune protein that kills bacteria, viruses and even cancer cells. Interleukin-2 is produced in the body when the body suspects it has been invaded by germs. It helps white blood cells multiply and mature to fight off infections and diseases. The FDA has approved the use of Interleukin-2 in the treatment of some forms of cancers.

Magnesium

Magnesium is needed for more than 300 biochemical reactions in the body. It helps maintain normal muscle and nerve function, keeps heart rhythm steady, supports a healthy immune system, and keeps bones strong. Magnesium also helps regulate blood sugar levels, promotes normal blood pressure, and is known to be involved in energy metabolism and protein synthesis.

Magnesium has been found to influence the body's utilization of Vitamin D in the following ways: Magnesium activates cellular enzymatic activity. In fact, all the enzymes that metabolize Vitamin D require magnesium.

Selenium

Selenium is a trace mineral that is essential to good health but required only in small amounts. Selenium is incorporated into proteins to make selenoproteins, which are important antioxidant enzymes. The antioxidant properties of selenoproteins help prevent cellular damage from free radicals. Free radicals are natural by-products of oxygen metabolism that may contribute to the development of chronic diseases such as cancer and heart disease

Selenium and zinc are essential minerals the body requires in order to produce antioxidant enzymes.

Zinc

Zinc is the most important mineral to add to your diet when you want to boost the immune system. Zinc boosts the immune system by helping to manufacture infection-fighting white bloods cells. Zinc also lowers the buildup of mucus.

Zinc is used by the body to form proteins and enzymes which help form new cells. It also frees Vitamin A which can get trapped in the liver (which keeps skin and tissue healthy and plays a part in bone growth).

Folic Acid

Folic acid is also known as Vitamin B9 or folate. It is an essential vitamin that is necessary for nearly every type of body function. Folic acid is used to make red blood cells, and also partners with other vitamins to catalyze your cell metabolism and the production proteins. An adequate supply of folate is critical to avoid cell mutation, tumor growth, and genetic disorders. Folate is more active in cells that are fast to grow and reproduce. An example of this is your blood. Your body doesn't make folic acid on its own so you have to get it either through food or nutritional supplements.

I took all of these as well as various herbs and tinctures including tincture of chaparral, a Native American remedy said to have a high antioxidant content, which can protect one against the cell damage leading to cancer. It may inhibit the growth of tumorous cancer cells. This was the nastiest tasting of all. It grows in the desert all around us and I had always believed it to be poisonous, but my doctor told me to drink an ounce of it every day. So I put it in a shot glass, pretended I was a saloon girl in an old wild-west film, and chugged it down first thing every morning. If that doesn't wake you up, nothing will. It is extremely bitter. Chaparral is known for stimulating the immune system. It is believed to protect against harmful effects of radiation and its greatest ability is moving the lymphatic system. This helps draw the harmful drugs and toxic chemicals out of the cells which is very beneficial for patients undergoing chemotherapy. You absolutely must consult your health care advisor if you choose to add this herb to your treatment regime.

My sister was very involved with organic gardening and homeopathic treatments so she called one of her friends and told her of my cancer. The friend immediately brewed up some Essiac tea, which is made from various herbs including slippery elm inner bark, Indian rhubarb root, burdock root, and sheep sorrel, known for over a hundred years as a cancer fighting herb. It is believed this tea boosts the immune system. I checked with my doctor as to whether or not I could take this and he said he didn't believe it would hurt me. It didn't taste good either, but not nearly as bitter as the chaparral. I actually began to like it so much that in the summer, I made it into iced tea and drank it throughout the day. You have to be very careful with this tea as it must be stored in glass bottles…no plastic. And it sometimes gets mold on it. You don't want to drink it then. I'd suggest researching this before trying it and ask your health care advisor about trying it.

The need for self-care is ever more prevalent today as the stresses of our competitive lifestyles take their toll on our bodies. There is a wealth of new scientific research supporting the use of nutritional alternatives in boosting the emotional and immune systems required to overcome diseases. With the right strategy, you can make the lifestyle changes necessary to become healthy and stay healthy. Do your homework! Then take action!

CHAPTER 7

Making Lifestyle Changes

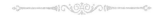

IN ADDITION TO ALL THE DIETARY CHANGES, THERE ARE OTHER important lifestyle changes which we can make to assist in boosting the immune system.

Exercise

We all need some form of physical exercise every day. Try a twenty-minute quick pace walk daily. Every other day, practice moderate strength training.

> *"Those who think they have no time for exercise will sooner or later have to find time for illness."*
>
> —EDWARD STANLEY
>
>

You need daily exercise to oxygenate the cells in your body. All my life, people told me that I needed to exercise. I personally don't like exercise so it was hard for me to grasp the concept that I needed to do it. Dr. Holcomb explained to me I needed to get on a bouncer and bounce up and down for 15 minutes a day to encourage the circulation of lymph and oxygen throughout my body. I understood him to say that without the exercise, my body would not function properly, and it wouldn't fight off the cancer. That got my attention.

Our bodies have a lymph system, which is a network made up of lymph vessels and lymph nodes. This network collects the fluid and debris in the body's tissue, outside of the bloodstream.

Lymph is the fluid that flows out from capillary walls to bathe the cells in the tissues of the body. It carries oxygen and other nutrients to those cells. It also contains white blood cells, which help fight infections. Waste products flow out of the cells and into the lymph. Lymph fluid can build up and cause swelling, if it isn't drained in some way.

Lymph vessels route the fluid through the lymph nodes which are located throughout the body. Lymph nodes work as filters for harmful substances. They contain immune cells that attack and destroy germs in the lymph fluid to help fight infection. Each lymph node filters fluid and substances picked up by the vessels that lead to it.

So, it seemed to me the lymph nodes have a purpose, should remain in my body, and I need to do all I can to assist them in circulating oxygen and supporting my immune system. If bouncing up and down on the bouncer for 15 minutes each day will keep the oxygen moving through my body, then I will bounce. Now, I do daily circuit training, walk, go to ballroom dance classes regularly and even bought a bicycle. This all assists in keeping the oxygen moving throughout the body.

It is also important for us to know our body's pH (potential hydrogen) levels because this is the measure of how acidic or alkaline a substance is and determines the body's ability to exchange oxygen. Our bodies can't fight diseases if our pH is not properly balanced.

Nobel Prize winner, Dr. Otto Warburg, discovered that cancer cells only thrive in a low oxygen state. When the body's cells and tissue are below pH levels of 6.5 – 7.0, they are considered acidic and lose their ability to exchange oxygen, thus cancer cells are able to thrive. When the pH level is above 7.0, your cells and tissue are considered to be in an alkaline state and cancer cells find it difficult to survive due to the high oxygen content. Alkaline tissue actually holds up to twenty times more oxygen than acidic tissue and prevents cancer cells, viruses, bacteria, and fungus from growing. In fact, in a pH of 8.0 or greater, they absolutely can't survive.

The most significant reason for a high acidic body environment is prolonged stress. This causes a depletion of adrenaline in the body's cells. It is the job of adrenaline to utilize glucose from the body's cells for energy for the body. Exercise helps deplete stress. Not only does it get oxygen into the system, it releases endorphins which help us better cope with stress. The increase in endorphins in our bodies leads to an enhancement of immune response.

Feelings of anger, hate, resentment, and grief create a drain on our adrenal system. These feelings need to be expressed and permanently released in order to prevent our bodies from returning to a lower adrenaline state, thus creating an acidic pH state.

Physical activity is great for expressing feelings and increasing your adrenaline. It is also good for our waistlines. If exercise has not been a part of your pre-cancer lifestyle, don't go wild now. Try something simple and easy, like walking.

Walking is probably the best exercise for maintaining health and fitness. Walk for about 20 minutes per day at a comfortable pace three times per week. Start out slow and increase your pace as you become more fit. Walk in a place where there are interesting sights, smells, and sounds so you will enjoy your time.

Wear a comfortable pair of sneakers or walking shoes, not running shoes. The shoe should have a low heel and a thick sole so as to cushion the foot from stones or holes in the road or path. The lighter the weight of the shoe, the better.

Other activities which aren't too strenuous and you might enjoy include bicycling, ballroom dancing, gardening, golf, swimming, or tennis. Be careful not to push yourself too hard, especially if you are over 45 or you have any history of illness, joint problems, or are on medication. Always talk with your doctor before beginning any exercise program.

If you want to rid yourself of cancer, exercise is imperative. For a long time, researchers have observed and communicated the positive effects of moderate exercise on the immune system. Recent research is revealing that women undergoing breast cancer treatment who exercise three or more times per week increase their immune cell counts to normal levels as well as improve their moods and their ability to more comfortably handle their feelings.

Don't create unrealistic expectations of yourself. If you didn't exercise before the cancer, undergoing a rigorous new exercise program could be detrimental. Start slow. The treatment you are having, your energy level, and your other life demands all play a part in how much energy you have. Do what you can and build up to more as your strength permits. There were days when I didn't want to exercise, but I found when I pushed myself a bit, I felt better. Stretching is a great form of exercise and is very helpful in the reduction of lymphedema, a condition sometimes caused by the removal of lymph nodes during cancer surgery which can leave that part of the body without a way to drain off excess fluids in the affected area.

Colonics

When the doctor told me that one of the most important things I needed to do to overcome my cancer would be to clean out my inside by having colonics ten days in a row, I was a bit uncomfortable. My apprehension was based on a lifetime of learned modesty and topics which were considered taboo. It turned out not to be uncomfortable or embarrassing at all. This process of cleansing the large intestine or colon with water from an external source makes sure your colon and the rest of the digestive system is in optimum working condition. The purpose of colonics is to remove toxic materials, to provide relief of intestinal stress, and to enhance appropriate function by stimulation of the intestinal muscles. If left un-cleansed, the colon and liver can accumulate toxins and wastes that deplete your energy and weaken the immune response.

After the initial cleansing, we cut back to three visits a month and increased the fiber in my diet. I have to admit, the colonics made me feel clean and light and encouraged me to make healthier eating choices.

Massage

A wonderful way to relieve stress is to get a massage a minimum of once a month. When your muscles are uptight, it is imperative you learn to relax. Massage not only relieves tension in the body, it soothes your anxiety, increases your circulation, provides human

> *"By cleansing your body on a regular basis and eliminating as many toxins as possible from your environment, your body can begin to heal itself, prevent disease, and become stronger and more resilient than you ever dreamed possible."*
>
> —DR. EDWARD GROUP III
>
>

contact, and most of all, improves healing. Many people feel they can't afford massage. I believe you can't afford NOT to get regular massages. If you don't have the cash, offer a "trade" of services. During my healing process, I was teaching at a college which offered a course in massage and the head of that department invited me to come in for a complimentary massage. It was so invigorating, I worked out a trade agreement with him for future massages, and have since continued with regular twice a week massages. This has made a positive difference in my life.

Dry Brushing

Another practice which I feel you will want to make a habit is dry brushing. This is a way to stimulate your organs to detox and it provides a gentle internal massage. Dry brushing assists in cleansing the lymphatic system, removing dead skin layers, strengthening the immune system, and stimulating the hormone and oil glands, as well as your circulation. Refer to the Appendix for a full explanation of dry brushing.

Rest

Sleep is absolutely necessary for you to regain your health. You must have sleep for your body to reach a state of harmony. What's missing in a stressed life is peace. Lack of peace causes sleeplessness. You know the amount of sleep you need to feel rested.

If you have trouble sleeping, try wearing yourself out physically. Work out, walk, run, or ride a bicycle. Stress is held in the muscles and you must use the muscles to be able to release the tension that is built up in them.

If your lack of sleep is caused by your mind going over all the problems of the day and all the things you must do tomorrow, create a bedtime ritual. Whether you choose meditating, yoga, or having a cup of tea is up to you. Turn off the television at a certain time, take a long, hot bath, cleanse your face, brush your teeth, put on fresh pajamas or nightie and crawl in bed. Read something positive or turn out the light and count your blessings. Following a regular routine gives your body and mind a gentle reminder that soon it will be time to relax and sleep.

Drinking alcohol can cause interrupted sleep. You may drink a lot and pass out early, but usually you'll awaken in a couple of hours and have difficulty falling back asleep. That's what happens to me when I have a bit too much wine.

When I am trying to wind down from the stresses of the day, I lie in bed and listen to my breathing. As my breathing slows down, I imagine it making a happy, humming sound. When I breathe in, it sounds like "ho" and as I breathe out, it sounds like "hum." As the breathing slows down, it sounds like "hoooooo, hummmmm." I find as I concentrate on my breath and the warm, soothing sound of "ho, hum," before long I am asleep. You might want to try it. I found it to be a great stress reducer.

Also, short naps in the daytime can be quite beneficial for the reduction of stress. This was quite difficult for me to do as I felt I had to be productive during working hours, but sometimes I'd get so tired, I felt I just couldn't go on, so I'd take a nap and in an hour or two, I'd be renewed and refreshed and could get more done than when I kept plugging along.

Journaling

A good way to find out what is working in your life and what is not working is to write down what is on your mind every day. Because it takes twenty-one days to change a habit, it is important to document the date when you decide to make a change and why it is that you want to make that change. Write in your journal each day, noting what you did that day to effect a desired change, what difficulties you encountered, and what you could do to overcome them. Most importantly, be sure to include your successes.

Write down what you eat, whether or not you exercised, when you rested and for how long, what you do, where you go, and what you are dealing with. Be honest. This is not for anyone else to read. It's for you to do an honest assessment of where you are right now. If you are to get well, you need to know where you are and what you must change to become healthy and whole again. If you are well, you need to understand how you helped your body get that way in order to maintain your healthy state.

At the end of every day, I record my daily "miracles" in my journal. Miracles are the way life responds to our wishes, dreams, desires, and visualizations. In the book, I also write my gratitude for what I have, the people I meet, and the things I experience. By writing in the book every day, we are reminding ourselves of the positive things that are happening and the very miracle of our lives.

I designed my own journal over a period of 20 years adapting it to life as my life changed. I found this was the perfect journal for me to use during the cancer as it has pages to assess if I'm keeping my life in balance, daily affirmations, questions to be answered about coping with life, an actual agreement with myself for how I will do things differently, a place for my bucket list, and peel and stick gold stars to use to reward myself daily as well as a place to write my miracles. If you would like your own copy of this journal, you can order one on my website www.judimoreo.com or call me at (702) 896-2228.

Use Color To Lift Your Spirits

You've probably noticed that certain colors have certain effects on your feelings and your moods. We feel different when we wear a bright color than we do when we wear a drab color. When we walk into a dimly lighted room, we feel different than we do when we walk into one that is brightly lighted.

Research shows that colors affect our emotional and physical health by easing stress, filling us with energy, and even alleviating pain and other physical problems. When we are not feeling well physically or emotionally, we should surround ourselves with colors in the "up" spectrum: yellow, orange, red, and violet. These have an energizing effect and can help relieve depression. Use blue to create a relaxing, peaceful, and calming effect, similar to the feeling you might get when you are in a place where you see and experience the blue sky and the ocean.

Green plants add a healing energy to a room and green foods, added to your diet, promote healing and growth.

Dr. Alexander Schauss, director of the American Institute for Biosocial Research in Tacoma, Washington, believes that when the energy of color enters our bodies, it stimulates the pituitary and pineal glands. This in turn affects the production of certain hormones, which in turn affect a variety of physiological processes. This explains why color has been found to have such a direct influence on our thoughts, moods, and behaviors.

Choosing to surround yourself with soothing, healing, happy colors can have a profound effect on your health.

You know your body better than anyone else. You have been with you all your life. You know how you feel when you've exercised, accomplished something creative, eaten a healthy meal, spent time outdoors or in a beautiful room or worn a gorgeous outfit in a color you love. This is the time to create the life you've always wanted, surround yourself with beautiful colors and things, travel to places you've always wanted to see, do the things you've wanted to do, and take care of yourself more than ever before. Stay focused on your health. Your body and your mind are always speaking to you. You must not be too distracted by life to listen.

CHAPTER 8

Reprogramming Your Mind

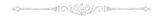

THIS CHAPTER MAY SEEM A BIT "WOO-WOO" TO SOME OF YOU, BUT I guarantee you, it is one of the most important chapters in the book. The practices I'm sharing here are crucial to your healing.

We got sick because something wasn't right in our lives. Whatever that something was, it caused us to have stress. It is a well-known fact that high levels of stress hormones suppress the immune system and inhibit the body's ability to defend and repair itself. In fact, many cancer centers and hospitals now offer stress reduction therapy along with conventional medical treatment for cancer patients. Meditation, visualization, yoga and other relaxation techniques are being recommended to boost the immune system and assist in fighting cancer.

You can enhance your immune system by doing things that make you happy and eliminating things that make you unhappy. Sounds simple enough, but it's not that easy.

Self-Talk

We all talk to ourselves…consciously or unconsciously. To some degree or another, most of us talk to ourselves in a negative fashion.

Many of us talk to ourselves worse than we would ever talk to someone else. In fact, about 70% of the negativity you and I hear every day comes out of our own mouths. We complain about our hair, our bodies, our clothing, our kids, our spouses, our other relatives, food, the traffic, the weather, and a multitude of other things. Take control of what you say. Think before you speak; eliminate negative statements from your dialogue. Don't talk about sickness or how bad you feel. Concentrate on your health. What felt good today?

Affirmations

Replace negative self-talk with positive self-talk, known as affirmations. These are positive statements said in the present tense that we repeat to ourselves in order to bring our minds to a state of consciousness where it accepts that which it is told.

To "affirm" means to "make firm." Make firm the loving, healing and positive thoughts you have about yourself and your life. Affirmations usually begin with "I am…." and are **always** stated in the present tense. Claim what you want as though you already have it. "I am healthy and happy," not "I don't want to be sick." The subconscious mind doesn't know the difference between real and imagined. It only knows what you tell it.

When you first start saying affirmations, your subconscious may want to argue with you. You may say, "I'm healthy and happy" and it will say, "No, you are not. You are sick." When you hear that little voice inside your head saying something negative to you, talk back to it. Say, "Thank you for sharing. Now go away." Then say something positive you know to be true about yourself. The Roman philosopher, Marcus Aurelius said, "Your life is what your thoughts make it." This is so true! That's why it is mandatory for you to control your thoughts, especially when you have been diagnosed with a life threatening disease.

Our thoughts create pictures in our minds. These pictures evoke feelings and emotions. Negative pictures evoke negative feelings and emotions, reminding us of all our disappointments and hurts. Before long they become so vivid, we re-live the pain and believe we got what we deserved. We may even believe we deserve to be sick.

Create a mental picture of yourself as a healthy, happy person. Look at all the good traits and characteristics you have. Tell yourself all the good things you want and need to hear. What you tell yourself will determine your self-image. This is why it's important to talk to yourself with love, kindness, and caring.

> "The difficult times are often the best teachers, and there is good to be found in all situations."
>
> —PAMELA OWENS RENFRO

What you believe to be true about yourself is what you make happen in your life. You view the world through your belief system. Since beliefs are usually formed as a result of what someone else told us about ourselves, our intelligence, our health, our diets, our possibilities, and our circumstances, we've learned to see the world through what we were taught by others. Don't you think it's about time you take charge of your own beliefs? Your self-concept is what determines your performance. You will always take the action that is consistent with your concept of yourself.

The only way you will change your outcome is to change the way you think. Your thoughts create your feelings. Your feelings direct your behavior. Your behavior brings about your results. You will not have different results in your life until you change your thinking. With affirmations, you gain the courage to do the things you'd like to do, increase your passion for life, and even take control of your emotions and your health. You must repeat your affirmations regularly for a period of no less than twenty-one days in order to override the belief system you now have in place.

I knew I had to live. I had things to do and people who depended on me. I wanted to live and I was willing to do whatever it took to live a healthy life.

How badly do you want to live a healthy life? Are you willing to do the work needed? Once you come to terms with the depth of your desires and have clarified your goals, it will be time to take action. Right now, you must sell yourself on the idea that you can and will make it happen. Reprogram your mind through your "self-talk." Tell yourself something along the lines of "I have the ability to get the information and knowledge I need," or "Every day in every way, I am getting healthier and healthier." Reminder — Repeat your statement a minimum of two times a day for twenty-one days. I sometimes repeat mine seven or eight times a day. I write them on Post-it notes and put them where I will see them...the car visor, the refrigerator, the bathroom mirror, and in my wallet.

Be sure to write out your affirmation statements before you start repeating them. In this way, you can be sure you have the self-talk worded in the best possible way for programming your mind for a successful outcome. When writing, emphasize gain rather than loss. Don't describe what you don't want. Instead, focus on what you do want. Write the statement so it creates a positive picture in your mind. "I am healthy and happy." Phrase it as though you are already there instead of, "I am going to be healthy and happy." When you say, "I am going to...," it puts the action out in the future somewhere. Make your affirmations short and easy to understand. Carry them with you. Read them over and over. If you repeat them enough, you will eventually believe them.

Robert Collier, one of our country's original self-help gurus said, "Any thought that is passed on to the subconscious often enough and convincingly enough is finally accepted."

In his book, *The Magic of Believing*, Claude Bristol tells us, "This subtle force of repeated suggestion overcomes reason. It acts directly on our emotions and our feelings, and finally penetrates to the very depths of our subconscious minds. It's the repeated suggestion that makes you believe."

So, begin each day with your affirmations. After awakening, in a very quiet, comfortable place where you won't be disturbed, clear your mind. You can do this by thinking of some place you love to spend time or a restful scene like green hills where you can hear a babbling brook off in the distance. Then think about all the things you have to be grateful for — your family, adequate food and shelter, freedom, the right to choose, etc. Remind yourself of the successes you have had in life — big and small, the obstacles you've overcome, and the love you've shared. Think about the strengths and characteristics that make you who you are. Then, tell yourself you will reach your next goal. Every morning, just after prayer, I do my affirmations. On the days I was working to overcome the cancer, my affirmations often sounded like this:

"I am alive and well. I am healing, fully and naturally. I am stronger. I am better. I am doing all the right things. I am eating healthy foods and exercising. I am grateful for so much. I am loved. With God, all things are possible. Together, we can do this. We are doing this."

If you would like, you are welcome to use mine until you make your own. Start today.

Say your affirmations again every night before going to sleep, any time you hear a negative statement from yourself or others, and any time you have doubts about achieving what it is you want.

Any time you start to feel depressed or negative, do it again. It's not possible to think two thoughts at the same time, so if you find yourself thinking a negative thought, change it to something positive. Review your accomplishments, strengths, and blessings. This act will push the negativity out of your mind.

Once something is recorded in the subconscious, it will stay there, replaying itself until you choose to displace it and diligently work to do so. Every statement you make to yourself has an effect on your subconscious, so be very careful about what you say.

Meditation

> *"Take time to let your thoughts drift, your muscles relax, and your dreams unfurl...*
>
> *Give yourself moments of absolute stillness to hear your wise inner voice and to heal."*
>
> —SUSAN SKOG

Meditation is a state of focused attention through which we emerge into an ever-increasingly clear awareness of reality. There are many different types of meditation: breath control, observation, imagery, and mantras. For me, meditation means I'm simply stopping my awareness of the world for the moment. My mind has a hard time stopping. It is constantly thinking and jumps from one thought to the next. In the beginning, when I tried not to think, I would think about why I wasn't able to not think. If this happens to you, it's okay. Just label your thoughts. When you have a thought, put it in a category. Before long, you'll see which thoughts you care to continue with and which ones you want to eliminate. It will be as if you are watching a movie. After a while, you'll get tired of the reruns and you'll come to a place of silence and light. This is such an awesome place to be. I've put a quick guide to meditation for your use in the Appendix of this book.

Visualization

Visualizing is imagining the outcome of something — what the future will be. Many of us used this skill when we were children. I've used it throughout my life and especially during the cancer period. You can use this same skill today. Imagine yourself being the healthy, happy person you want to become. Shakespeare said, "Assume a virtue if you have it not." In other words, act the part. "Oh sure," you say. "That sounds easy. Who are you kidding?" I can just hear you.

I'm not kidding. The subconscious part of our minds causes us to feel and act in agreement with what we imagine to be true about ourselves and our environment. When we realize our behaviors are a result of the images and beliefs our minds create, we free ourselves to use our imaginations as though our thoughts are reality. If we see ourselves performing a certain way, our subconscious mind perceives we are actually performing that way. As I mentioned before, the subconscious doesn't know the difference between what is real and what is imagined. It only knows what we tell it. We can think ourselves into health, success, and prosperity by concentrating on the good we have now and focusing on a positive future. Whatever thoughts you hold in your conscious mind give direction to your subconscious. Whatever you impress on your subconscious mind will be what you experience in your life. William James, the father of American psychology, said, "The power to move the world is in your subconscious mind."

Whenever we create something, we create it first in our minds as thoughts. As a young girl, my mother taught me to sew. First, we would go to the fabric store and select a picture from the pattern book of the garment I would like to have. We would get the pattern and read the instructions on the back to see how much fabric it would take to make this particular garment as well as what other notions we would need. Then we would go through the store and select a fabric, trim, such as lace or ribbon, some buttons, as well as thread and a zipper. I would get so excited. I could see that garment made with that fabric before it was even cut out. I could see me wearing it and how happy I was going to be. Then we would go home, lay the pattern on the fabric, pin the pattern down, cut the fabric, pin it together and sew it up. In hardly any time at all, I would have a new dress! In fact, the more excited I was about it, the sooner the dress would get finished.

That's how visualization works in your life. First, you get the picture in your mind. Get clear on the outcome you desire. Vividly imagine it. Imagine how you are going to look, how you are going to feel, what supplies or resources you will need to have, and what lifestyle changes you will make. You must be able to see it in your mind in complete detail and feel it in your very being. If you will consciously hold this picture in your mind, the imagination which is based in the subconscious part of your mind, will start working on the "how to" part of the equation and bring you to a logical approach for making that picture become a reality. Once you have the vision, you are ready to start making your action plan, exploring your possibilities, and setting your goals.

Whether it is a creative endeavor like sewing or a stressful event in life, like being diagnosed with cancer, you can prepare yourself for it by imagining the scenario and seeing the outcome the way you want it to be. Imagine what it will be like to be well and happy. Imagine what you will do when the doctor says you are cancer free. You are conditioning your mind, which causes the rest of you to act confidently in this particular situation. If you allow yourself to imagine what it will be like to be sick, how you will feel when you lose your hair, and how you are going to die, then that is likely what is going to happen.

Your imagination is where your creativity begins. When we imagine something, we can actually cause it to become reality. It is an idea and then we start to think of it as a possibility. You've seen science fiction movies that had plots so far "out there" no one would ever believe they could be real. Yet, within a few years "science fiction" became "science fact" as those scenarios became reality; man orbited the earth and subsequently walked — and even played golf — on the moon.

Decide what you want to do, believe you can do it, make a plan of how you will do it, and then act on your plan. Marcus Aurelius said, "If the mind of man can conceive an idea and believe it, the man can achieve it." If we can create the image in our minds, we can produce the physical manifestation in our lives, even if such an image has never existed before! When you visualize something, you are establishing new patterns in your brain, the same as if you were actually doing what you are visualizing. You are directing your brain to give you the result you want to achieve. When you plan your new healthy life, it works the same way. You are visualizing each day. As you go through your activities, you may have to adjust and modify your actions in order to achieve the results you want.

Imagine every detail of your new, healthier life. Many people use their imagination in the opposite way. Unsuccessful people are usually unmotivated and unexcited about where they are going. It doesn't really matter what happens; their minds are conjuring up all the things that can go wrong, won't happen, or will disappoint them. There are even some of you who are thinking as you read this, "Oh, what a bunch of bunk. This stuff doesn't work." If those are your thoughts, guess what! That's what will be true for you and that proves it works. You'll think it won't work and so it won't. You get what you think. My suggestion to you is, "Just try it. You have nothing to lose by trying it...and a whole, new, healthy life to gain."

Don't buy into negativity! Get rid of mental limitations. You can do it simply by imagining and focusing on what it is you **do** want, instead of what you **don't** want. Whatever you focus on is what you get. Remember, if you focus on what you don't want, you'll get that just as surely as if you focus on what you want.

The subconscious part of your mind ignores the words "not" and "don't" and translates the message the same as if you had asked for what you don't want. So if you say, "I am not going to be sick," the subconscious hears, "I am going to be sick" and directs your conscious mind to do exactly that. Instead, say, "I am well and happy," or "Every day in every way, I am getting better and better."

Miracles happen ...if you believe they will. I know. I've experienced them. I am well and happy. I intend to stay that way. When I go for my bi-monthly blood tests, my oncologist often says, "Well, how's our miracle lady today?" Several times, he's said, "I'm so proud of you."

We all visualize — often. We consider the future, and envision it either positively or negatively. Our problems occur when we negatively visualize — imagining a future of lack, loneliness, and despair. Take a moment and visualize a positive outcome. Imagine yourself healed, happily alive, thriving, loving and loved. Use as many of your senses as you can. See, feel, hear, taste, and smell your happy, healthy future. It will help you to cut out words and pictures of all the things you want to be, do, and have — such as a healthy body — and paste these words and pictures in a journal. Or paste them on a big piece of construction paper and tack it on the wall where you can see it every day. I put mine in my journal because I look in that book every day. You may need to start your visualization exercises slowly — a minute or so at first. That's okay. Then build — visualization by visualization, day by day — imagining your positive future for longer and longer periods of time. Soon your present will be the positive future you are imagining now.

CHAPTER 9

Adjusting Your Attitude

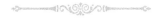

BELIEVE YOU WILL SURVIVE. CANCER DOES NOT MEAN YOU ARE GOING to die. There are millions of cancer survivors in this world. You can be one of them. Make up your mind you are going to do everything you can to boost your immune system enabling it to fight the cancer. Decide you are going to get well and then take the necessary steps.

Three stressors which could be affecting you are loss of control, loss of hope, and a feeling of aloneness. If you can address and overcome these, you give power to your immune system and affect its ability to fight off cancer.

The cancer experience was unlike any other I had ever had. First, I was in shock…then disbelief. Then I was angry. Real angry, about the unfairness of life. Then came the doubts and questions.

> *"A spiritually toxic attitude after a cancer diagnosis can make your life a living hell."*
>
> —ANONYMOUS

Did I bring this on myself? Or was it the gynecologist who put me on hormone replacement therapy for all those years?

I tried to stay calm, but I was very concerned as to what would happen to my sister if I wasn't around to take care of her. Then there were all the different recommendations from the doctors, friends, and family. I still had to work and I was trying to stay positive and motivational. After all, I am a motivational speaker and writer. Some days it was overwhelming. In fact, in the beginning, most days...it was overwhelming.

What I didn't realize was that I had time. When the surgeon said you need surgery tomorrow, I did it. Isn't that what you are supposed to do...what the doctor tells you? If I had it to do over, I wouldn't have done it so fast. I would take more time. We don't get cancer over night and we can certainly take the time to make our decisions based on information, knowledge, and the assurance we are doing the right thing. This hurry up and do something panic is not based on fact; it is based in fear. Our minds start to create scenarios when we are faced with the unknown.

What should we do when we start to panic? Observe. Observe yourself, your emotions, and what's going on around you. Separate in your mind who you are from the panic you are feeling. Simply watch your emotions and let them go. Visualize yourself as a competent person who can make the right decisions. Say prayers of thanksgiving. "Thank you, God, for giving me the intelligence and the power to make the right decision for all concerned in this situation. Thank you, God, for giving me a long and healthy life."

Do you believe things happen for a reason? Or are you caught up in your "poor me" routine? Attitude is one of the few things in life over which we have complete control. In fact, in times like these, it is probably the only thing. We can discipline our minds to take possession of our thoughts. I know it's not easy. In fact, it is very hard to be positive when you are scared and overwhelmed.

American psychologist, William James, once said, "As you think, so shall you be." These words resonated with me, and I worked daily to discipline my mind in order to maintain a positive focus. When I allowed my mind to be filled with fear and doubt, that's when I scared away any chance of the healthy life I so desperately wanted to live. I had to control my attitude.

You may be asking yourself, "What has attitude got to do with taking control of my health?

Our attitude is our outward expression of our feelings. Our thoughts create our feelings, and our feelings usually determine our behavior. Remember, when we improve our thoughts, we improve our feelings, which in turn, improves our behavior, and leads directly to improved results.

> *"You do what you have to do to get through today, and that puts you in the best place tomorrow."*
>
> —OPRAH WINFREY

It is important to process our thoughts so they move us forward. If we remain positively focused on the good health we want in our lives, we won't have time to get sidetracked by things and circumstances we don't want.

Why is it, for many of us, when a difficult experience comes our way, we interpret it as a hardship? When things happen to us, we can choose to believe they happened for the best. We can discover opportunities in even the most difficult of situations if we are willing to look for them. It is what we think about each experience that determines how we respond to it. If we think, "This is a disaster," it will be. On the other hand, if we think, "There's an opportunity in here somewhere," and look for it, we will most certainly find it.

Learn More

Acquire as much knowledge as possible about the situation you are going through. Research the dis-ease, the treatments, the cures, the doctors, and nutritional programs. Talk to other people who have been in similar circumstances to yours and find out about their treatments and their results. Find out what the side effects of their treatments were. The more you know, the more confident you will feel. Confident thinking leads to a positive attitude, which leads to successful outcomes.

Identify the Pitfalls

Identify what could go wrong with your plans. If you know the possible pitfalls, it's easier to work around them. Unknown factors breed fear. Once you expose fears to the light of day, evaluate them, and start exploring ways to overcome them, they will no longer seem so scary.

We naturally experience fear when we step out of our comfort zones. It is one of the ways we protect ourselves. When we have fear, we are usually more cautious. Examine your fears. What is it you are actually afraid of? I wasn't afraid to die. I was afraid to be sick. Once I realized that, I was able to be more courageous in my treatment options.

Have you done your homework? Have you looked at all your options? What's motivating you to take the action you are taking? Is it your decision or someone else's? Do you feel in control or out of control? Do you have all the information you need? If not, why not?

Take positive steps toward a healthier you. Sell yourself on doing whatever it is that you need to do.

Learn Positive Self-Talk

Self-talk is the conversation you have with yourself. We've discussed this before, but it's important to remember that your mind will believe whatever you tell it if you tell it often enough and with conviction. Our minds have such power. If we tell them that we are strong and healthy, they will say, "Yes," and start to work on taking us down the path to a successful outcome. If we tell them we are weak and scared, they will also say "Yes," and take us down the path to fear and doubt.

Ask yourself, "Am I reacting to life or living my life in a proactive manner? Am I so busy being caught up in what is wrong now that I'm not working out a plan for my successful outcomes? Am I allowing my life to be governed by outside forces or am I choosing to live my life in accordance with my own decisions? Do I have important goals and dreams that I am committed to, or am I creatively avoiding life by allowing this dis-ease to have its way with me?

Surround Yourself With Positive People

There are people who will try to convince you that you shouldn't try any of this. They will tell you it's ridiculous, that it won't work. Don't believe them. At this point, you must try anything that resonates with you that it might possibly work. Surround yourself with people who support you and believe you will be well and whole again.

Close your mind to the negativity of those around you. Negativity is a virus and it is catching. Make yourself immune to it by understanding that no one else can make you feel anything. No one else can make you angry. No one else can make you sad. No one else can hurt your feelings. Unless you allow them to! You choose how you react and respond to situations and what others say and do. They can trigger old feelings from the past, but they can't determine how you feel or how you behave. How you react or respond is up to you! Change your thinking about the situation, and you control your behavior.

I had to stay away from people who were negative. I needed all my strength to stay positive and focus forward on my health and my new, better life. It wasn't easy. About a month into the cancer experience, my sister died suddenly. That was such a shock. I had to arrange for her funeral and deal with her estate. I went to stay at her farm while I went through her things and sorted out everything. I came home for one weekend and, while I was home, the farm was burglarized. It was devastating. I called the sheriff. The sheriff's department did an investigation and found that it was a neighbor who had done the burglarizing, so they seized as much as they could find and brought back truckloads of "stuff" which now had to be sorted all over again. In addition, a long process of identifying my sister's things, pressing charges, going to court and testifying began. There were days when I felt I couldn't go on. I would talk to God. I asked Him why...why was I being given so much to deal with at one time. I was so fortunate to have some incredible friends and some wonderful neighbors who came to my rescue, supported me, cooked for me, changed the locks, and generally were "there" for me. It feels so good when someone says, "I am here for you," and they really mean it.

Laugh, and Laugh Some More

> *"A good laugh and a long sleep are the best cures in the doctor's book."*
>
> —IRISH PROVERB

Laughter is one of the most healing activities around. Whatever it is that makes you laugh, do it. Laugh a lot. Watch every funny movie you can get your hands on. Hang out with friends who are happy and make you laugh. Go to comedy shows, rent a video, buy a comedy cd or dvd, read a funny book, ask your friends to call you with anecdotes, stories, and jokes. Sometimes, we laugh just because someone else is laughing. It's contagious.

It's good to laugh about things during illness. It makes us feel more alive. Laughter, like exercise, releases endorphins (the body's natural pain killers.) Even in the midst of pain, we can often find things to laugh about. At one point, when we were cleaning up my sisters farm, my friend, Charlotte, pulled a bag out of a shelf. It ripped and out flew a wooden snake. It looked so real, she screamed and screamed. When we discovered it was fake, we had such a good laugh. Actually, it was hysterical to even think about us two city slickers with our styled hair and fake fingernails cleaning out the barn with 30 years worth of storage. Every time we pulled a box down from the rafters and rat excrement fell into our hair, we launched into peals of laughter.

As early as the 13th century, surgeons used humor to distract patients from pain. In 1979, there appeared to be a real breakthrough when Norman Cousins wrote the book, *Anatomy of an Illness*, in which he credited watching comedic movies and laughter for curing himself of a serious illness with years of prolonged pain.

For people who have been diagnosed with a life threatening disease, it may seem odd to find humor when facing such a serious event. Remember, there is a fine line between tragedy and comedy. Seeing humor in your situation, your reaction to your situation, and even your memories about your dis-ease can be healing. When you are laughing, you aren't thinking negative thoughts. You are boosting your immune system, improving mental functions such as alertness, memory, and creativity, and inducing positive changes in your body. Sometimes, you'll feel better for hours after only a few minutes of laughter. Because laughter helps us relax, it often reduces stress and tension and produces an overall sense of well-being. There's a lot of truth in the old adage, "Those who laugh...last."

Be Grateful for Your Gifts

Every night, when you lay your head on your pillow, say thank you for at least two things in your life for which you are grateful. One night as I drifted off to sleep, I caught myself thinking, "I'm so happy." Then I wondered, "When was the last time I felt this way?" My healthier body and new energy, as well as my awareness of how fortunate I am to be alive, gave me a whole new sense of gratitude.

On those sometimes difficult nights — when you are laying there thinking about the things you haven't done, you still need to do, you could have said, you shouldn't have said, you don't have, or wish you did - concentrate on two people, traits, or things that happened which are a blessing to you. Think about what you have, instead of what you don't. Focus on what you are, instead of what you aren't. As Reverend Robert Schuller has often said, "Obstacles are seldom the same size tomorrow as they are today. Today's responsibilities are tomorrow's possibilities."

Maintaining Your New, Positive Attitude

Even the most successful people have experienced periods when they have been confused, disillusioned and discouraged. Yet, they have overcome trials and tribulations to achieve triumph and victory because they chose the right attitude. When we feel discouraged and stressed, when life seems intolerable, even meaningless, when our lives are not going the way we want, and when events are taking place so fast we don't know the questions, never mind the answers, doesn't it make sense we should take control of our thoughts, so that we, too, can triumph?

Life comes in a series of challenges. Certainly, a diagnosis of a life threatening disease is a challenge...a big one. The attitude with which we chose to perceive challenges and the mindset with which we face them determines whether our lives are rewarding or not.

CHAPTER 10

Building a Positive Support System

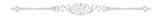

RELATIONSHIPS AFFECT YOUR HEALTH. WE ARE CONSTANTLY interacting with other people. Whether or not we are getting along with the important people in our lives determines, to a large extent, the quality of our lives. Associate with positive, supportive people. Invest time in relationships which are nourishing. A strong, positive support team is vital, but so are positive relationships in every area of your life.

Be brave enough to ask for and accept the help of others. It's a human and courageous thing to do. Gather your friends, family, and co-workers into a support system. You need to know that others care and if you tell them what you need, they will help. Remember, others don't know what to do for you unless you tell them what you need. If someone asks you, "What can I do?" perhaps all you need to say is, "Hold my hand." The healing power of touch can't be overestimated. Maybe you'd like to have someone stay overnight and sit up and talk. You aren't too old to have a slumber party. Neighbors can be wonderful. Invite one or two over and have a tea party. Even your telephone can be a marvelous support tool. Call old friends.

Call someone you haven't seen in a long time. Call someone you'd like to see. Call someone you need to apologize to and do it. Or call someone who needs to apologize to you and tell him that you forgive him. (But only if you do!)

Seek out others who have been through what you have been through or something similar. Their support can be invaluable. People who have survived similar circumstances can provide support and guidance — and are proof that you, too, will survive. There are many organizations and support groups dedicated to serving others. Look in the Yellow Pages or go on the internet and Google "cancer organizations."

When we experience cancer, we often start to re-evaluate our lives. Then we begin to re-prioritize and often discover what really is important to us and what isn't.

Support groups give us a safe place to discuss our fears, feelings, and expectations. They are also a place of information exchange. Often, this helps us clarify what is important to us and we may learn how to be kinder to ourselves. Sometimes, we need to sift through our feelings about situations, people, and happenings in our lives in order to figure out what means the most to us. Support groups make us feel connected and when we realize we are not alone, somehow that helps reduce the stress of having the illness.

You may want to hire someone to stay with you or do things for you. Some people are so good at comforting others, they do it as a profession. Individuals who go into the health care field are usually caring people who can and will help others heal. These include professional caretakers, naturopaths, chiropractors, clinical psychologists, homeopaths, exercise and fitness trainers, massage therapists, nutritionists, ministers, psychiatrists, and stress management counselors.

Reading about the experiences of others can be helpful, too. I read every book I could find which had been written about cancer. I especially appreciated the ones where people shared their own stories about their cancer experiences. I even explored the treatments they talked about and checked out clinics and doctors mentioned.

Your job is to do whatever it takes to get and stay healthy. You must eat right, take your vitamins, get your exercise, rest, do something creative, play, and pamper yourself. Get massages, manicures, pedicures. Have your hair done. Get up every morning, fix your hair, put on your makeup, and dress for the day...even if you are staying home and relaxing. Live as though you are well, not as though you are an invalid. Take an art class, a dance class, or join a book club. It doesn't have to be expensive, there are a number of community associations, continuing education programs, and church outreach programs that offer all sorts of fun, creative activities. MAKE time for yourself. Life goes on. Some of us have to work and take care of our families, but we also need and deserve to do things which make us feel as though we are living...not dying.

Sometimes, it's difficult to keep a positive attitude, especially when you have people around you who are telling you what you should do, could do, and what they would do.

You are in control of your life, your body, your mind, and your well-being. Take charge of your relationships. Learn to say "No" to anything which doesn't promote your health and to anyone who doesn't support you in creating a stress free, healthy life style. Don't be surprised if others don't understand what you said or take things wrong. One man asked me about dating him at that time, and I told him it would be a difficult time to start a relationship. He later told someone I refused his offer to drive me to doctor appointments and to investigate clinics. That was not my understanding of his offer at all. Miscommunication happens, even when we are in the best of health, so we can't expect it not to happen when we are not well.

I was surprised and empowered by the support of other friends who absolutely believed I was making a mistake by not doing the chemo and radiation, yet in spite of their beliefs said, "It is your decision and I'll support you through it." I was even more surprised when a colleague's wife, whom I had only met once before, showed up at my home with half a dozen quarts of various homemade soups. What an incredibly thoughtful thing to do! Especially because she had made sure the ingredients were included in my list of things I could eat.

> *"We're lucky there are people placed in our paths to guide us, protect us, and touch our lives so we can get through it all... one day at a time."*
>
> —JULIA ESCOBAR
>
>

Loving relationships with friends, employees, and clients were what got me through the tough times. Cancer taught me to give up "toxic" relationships. It also taught me to speak up and tell people when I thought they were not treating me properly or not respecting me or my wishes.

I needed someone with whom I could be totally honest about what I was feeling, what I was thinking, and what I was considering without any judgment or criticism. I was fortunate to have two friends with whom I could share all of these things. These two people were by my side through it all...the good days and the bad. I will forever be grateful for their support.

Do you have someone with whom you can share your innermost secrets and feelings? Do you have a network of people who will support you? You might want to make a list of the most important relationships in your life. Are they serving you? Do you enjoy being with them? Are you interested in them as well as wanting them to be interested in you? Do you love them and feel loved by them? If not, you may want to highlight any relationships that need to be put on hold. Is there any reason to continue the relationship? If so, what can you do to improve it?

If a relationship is painful, eliminate it or change the way you think about it. If your feelings are hurt, so is your physical being. Eliminate "toxic" relationships. That includes friends, family, business associates, and doctors. If you are not comfortable… if you don't feel as though you are being treated with respect, honored and accepted for who you are or your thoughts and feelings are not being taken seriously, move on. You don't have to be taken for granted by anyone. This may mean some of the people who are now in your life must go.

Use your energy for healing yourself…not for dealing with the negativity of others. You must take responsibility for your own health.

If you have received a diagnosis of cancer or any other life changing illness, you must become your first priority…not your spouse, not your children, not your friends, not your job. YOU and your health are the most important things you have to deal with right now. All too often, we not only allow others to take us for granted, we do it to ourselves, putting "responsibilities," previous commitments, and relationships before our need to care for our bodies, minds, and souls.

Once you are well, there will be people who disappeared from your life who will suddenly reappear. Be very careful when allowing these people back into your life. Take the time to examine what your relationship was like before your illness. Was it supportive or was it negative and stressful? Did these people consider your needs? Or, were they only there for what you could do to help them? Did you look forward to events in which you knew they would be participating? Or, did you dread the time you would have to spend with them? You have the right to determine whether or not this is a relationship that contributes to your health and well being. If it doesn't, you have the responsibility to yourself to step back or walk away completely.

One of the most important relationships you have is the one you have with yourself. In the *Bible*, it says to "Love Thy neighbor as Thy self." It does not say to "Love Thy neighbor **instead** of Thy self." You can't expect others to treat you with respect if you don't respect yourself. Love yourself enough to be gentle with yourself. Talk kindly to yourself. Treat yourself with respect and love. Care for yourself. Eat the right foods. Rest when you feel you need rest. When others are not available to you, hug yourself. The most healing touch may be gently caressing yourself. If a part of you hurts, gently touch it and tell it, "I am here for you. I love you."

CHAPTER 11

Nourishing Your Soul

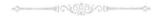

OVERCOMING CANCER REQUIRES THE PATIENT'S FULL PARTICIPATION. Only God knows how much time you have to live and He gives you the power to improve your potential for survival. As with all the other subjects I have taught in my lifetime, I say to you now, "Focus forward." Keep your thoughts and your sights on your goal. What is it going to take to heal? For me, it meant changing my diet, my exercise routine, and my periods of rest. It meant doing whatever it took to lower my stress levels. It meant sticking ever so much closer to my belief in and practices of visualization, affirmations, meditation, and most of all, prayer. I stayed focused on wellness and ridding my body of the cancer. I chose to live my life to the fullest. I listed the things I still want to do in life and I got about doing them. Somehow, this cancer was a catalyst to my finding inner peace, learning that most of the things in life about which I had worried really didn't warrant that kind of time or feeling, and now that I am on the other side, I have much more confidence and feel happier than I have ever felt before.

I believe this was a wake-up call from God. He was saying to me, "Why have you chosen a life in which you work extremely long hours and don't enjoy the journey? This was not what I had in mind for you."

My naturopath suggested I might want to take up some artistic endeavor, and even though I believed I had no talent for drawing or painting, I signed up for a watercolor art class. It was in one of those art classes that it hit me. "I am really enjoying this. I'm doing something I truly love. It is similar to meditation. It feels almost spiritual. I'm actually showing love to myself." Painting nourishes my soul. And I discovered I really did have a talent for it. One of my paintings recently won "Best of Show" in a local gallery art show.

William James once said, "The greatest discovery of our generation is that human beings, by changing their inner attitudes of mind can change the outer aspects of their lives."

Man doesn't create his power of thought. He uses it. He can either use it in the right way or the wrong way. God's truth and God's laws are always with us. It is up to us to recognize and use this power to bring good into our lives and the lives of those around us, as well as the world at large.

There is a system and a rhythm to the universe. It's God's rhythm. Day follows night. Night follows day. First comes winter, followed by spring, then summer, and autumn. Then we return to winter. It is our job to get into the rhythm of the universe. God wants us to be healthy, happy, and live a good life. It is up to us to remember and accept that.

The law of cause and effect tells us we can change the effect only by changing the cause. If we are thinking negative thoughts, we are going to get negative results. When you keep doing the same old thing in the same old way, it's not only called insanity...it's called pure stubbornness. If you want different results or a different effect, you must change the cause. I can't tell you how many people I know who have been through a cancer experience and then change nothing. They continue to eat the same way. They don't take supplements. They don't exercise. They don't practice visualization, prayer, or meditation. Then, when the cancer shows its nasty head again, they are devastated. Usually, they aren't surprised, because they expected it to come back. You get what you expect.

Once you understand and accept this, it will change your life. As we live our lives, we experience various degrees of consciousness. Whatever we have experienced thus far might have been experienced differently, if only we had understood that our expectations produced the results we achieved. If you want to grow strawberries, don't plant turnip seeds. If you want love in your life, don't plant hate. If you want wellness, do what will make you well.

> *"When you recover or discover something that nourishes your soul and brings joy, care enough about yourself to make room for it in your life."*
>
> —JEAN SHINODA BOLEN

Love heals. When we show love to ourselves and to others, we are taking positive action. Whenever we feel fear, we are actually experiencing a negative void — an absence of love. Focus on loving yourself because it will heal you. When you feel love, it will be easier to give love to others. Love doesn't mean you take some huge action. It means you focus on the positive and the good traits, how you might help another person, and how you might help yourself. Wellness comes when we are feeling emotionally and spiritually strong. These are a result of love.

> *"The soul always knows what to do to heal itself. The challenge is to silence the mind."*
>
> —CAROLINE MYSS

Love is a necessary ingredient to a happy, successful, joyous, creative, and productive life. Love is more important than knowledge. You can love yourself, even when you have cancer. You are you. Cancer is not a part of you. I refused to ever acknowledge it was mine. It was not "my" cancer. It was "the" cancer. I often hear cancer patients refer to their illness as "my cancer." Why would you want to claim it? Thank it for coming to you and showing you that changes need to be made and then release it. Let it go. Tell it to go. Cancer is not the enemy. It is a result of your dis-ease. Find out what is causing the dis-ease in your life and love yourself through it. One woman asked me, "Have you painted your cancer?" I could only respond with, "Why would I do that? It was never mine." Since she didn't answer me, I had to assume she had no good reason for her question.

Forgive yourself for whatever it is that you are feeling guilty or emotional about. Forgive others for the hurts they have caused. Forgiveness is the choice we make to change our perceptions of things, situations, and people and release the effects of toxic emotions. Forgiveness will help you find peace. If you switch your focus from fear, anger, and blame to forgiveness, you will find that you will feel more love, and healing begins.

Let's face it, we are harder on ourselves than we are on others. And, we are harder on ourselves than others would ever be. Listen to how we talk to ourselves sometimes. "I'm so stupid. I'm so dumb. I should have known better. I should have done better." We say things like, "You might know this would happen to me." Or, "Things never go well for me." Or even, "God is punishing me." Get rid of this kind of condemnation talk. It causes you to feel unworthy and sabotage any success or hope of getting well again. Just because you did something or said something at some time in your life that you feel guilty about or someone else did or said something for which you feel shame or resentment, it doesn't mean you are unworthy and deserve to have cancer.

Once you are in the negativity habit, it's not easily changed. But, it can be done. Practice your affirmations. Remember, you can't think two thoughts at the same exact time, so practice forgiving yourself. If you believe God is punishing you (which I don't believe), then ask Him for His forgiveness. Whenever, you hear one of these negative statements chattering away in your brain, tell it to "Stop." Actually say, "Stop!" aloud and correct it with a positive affirmation. It will take work, but good results come from disciplined thoughts and behaviors.

Why do we sometimes project blame for our limitations upon God? It is not God who limits us. It is our ignorance of the consciousness which God has given us. We need to boost ourselves up to greater wisdom, guidance, and self-expression. If you will take the time every day to sense the presence of God, you will pass from fear into faith. Start today by giving yourself permission to have faith and belief in order to regain your health.

Don't misunderstand. Faith by itself is not the answer to all that is wrong. While we rely on faith for guidance and comfort, it is our actions that produce results. We must act on the love and the peace that come from being connected to God. We can sit on a mountaintop and contemplate God and believe in our healing, but unless we take the necessary steps, nothing happens.

Realize, too, you are not responsible for the words and behaviors of others. People are people and they don't all do and say what we expect or desire. We don't have to approve of them, just accept them as they are. What is that old saying? "Forgive them for they see not what they do."

Life will be much easier when we learn to accept ourselves and others, accept that things don't always go as we think they should, and people don't always behave as we wish they would. All of us are imperfect in some way. Often, when we are diagnosed with a life threatening disease, we realize that many of the things we previously got so worked up about weren't really important at all. Forgiveness is easier when we realize the relative unimportance of the event. Amazingly, many people heal after they have learned to forgive. What a shame we couldn't have learned it earlier.

Think about this. If you are truly living in the "now," you aren't dragging along memories of past hurts and mistakes. Why do so many of us use up today with thoughts of yesterday? It's over. It's done. We can't change it. We can only go forward and do better. Let go of judgment. Let go of bitterness. Forgive.

Learn to love your life. Be grateful for who you are and what you have. Tell God thank you for the things that are going right in your life. We have so many blessings, and the majority of us take them for granted. Even when you have cancer, you have much to be thankful for. Do you have a home? A family who loves you? Friends? Pets? Good medical care? Insurance? Transportation to and from your treatments? Have you stepped outside and truly appreciated the fresh air, the sky, the trees, the flowers, the birds, and the grass? Have you thanked God for His presence?

Don't let yourself get so wrapped up in your illness that you stop being grateful. Yes, I understand our cancer journeys are filled with uncomfortable treatments, painfully long waits in doctor's offices, feelings of fear, despair, and even pain. We sometimes fall back into habits of complaining and allowing ourselves to be miserable. Stop! Get back on track. Say, "Thank you, God, for today."

CHAPTER 12

Continuing On

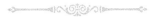

THE BODY, MIND, AND EMOTIONS HAVE ENORMOUS WISDOM. THEY know how to heal themselves and the amount of time they will need to do it. We must give them what they need in order to heal. Nature is on your side and is a powerful ally.

Reactions to the diagnosis of a life threatening disease takes place in three distinct-yet overlapping stages. They are:

- Shock/denial/numbness
- Fear/anger/depression
- Understanding/acceptance/moving on

The first stage of recovery is shock/denial/numbness:

- We can't believe or comprehend what has happened to us
- The mind denies the illness
- Often the first words out of our mouths after hearing the diagnosis are "Oh, no" or "Not me."
- We may shift back and forth between belief and disbelief that this is happening to us
- Shock and numbness set in

The second stage of recovery is fear/anger/depression:

- Feeling helpless, fearful, empty, irritable, angry, despairing, pessimistic, or depressed are all reactions which may happen when we are diagnosed with a life threatening disease.

- It's okay to feel all of these or to feel nothing.

- We may experience a loss of hope, motivation, energy or concentration.

- Our appetite, sleep patterns, and sexual desire may change.

- We may be more fatigued or prone to errors.

- Any and all of these emotions can be expected. It's a part of the healing process.

The third and final stage of recovery is understanding/acceptance/ moving on:

- It has happened. It is real.

- We understand and have accepted that we are experiencing a dis-ease.

- Our bodies are healing.

- Our minds accept that life will never be the same again.

- We move into a new chapter of our lives.

- The healing process has a beginning, a middle, and no end. We must live a new lifestyle. Our task is to make the journey from devastating diagnosis to eventual gain as rapidly, smoothly, and courageously as possible.

Once the doctor says you are in remission, cancer free, or even when the doctor says your cancer marker numbers are below the average person walking around, you must remember you are not an average person. You are a survivor and you must continue with the practices that made you well.

It's easy to fall back into old habits. It's easy to think if we eat a little bit of sugar, drink a couple of martinis or glasses of wine, or put foods we eliminated back into our diet, it will be okay. It will NOT be okay. You must stay with what got you well in order to stay well. It is not a cure. It is a lifestyle.

Once you have overcome the challenges of dealing with the "reality" of cancer, you have reached a place on your journey where you must make decisions about how you will live the rest of your life. If you are to maintain your new found health and vitality, you can't return to the habits that contributed to your illness.

No one is ever truly cancer free. All of us walk around with potential cancer cells in our bodies all of the time. While cancer is the irregular growth of abnormal cells, there are many lifestyle choices that are factors in that growth including attitudes, nutrition, exercise, spirituality, and associations. You remedied the illness because you discovered a way to correct what caused it. Going back to old habits, old stresses, and your old

> *"Your body cannot heal without play. Your mind cannot heal without laughter. Your soul cannot heal without joy."*
>
> —CATHERINE FENWICK
>
>

diet will not keep you from experiencing the illness again. You MUST maintain the new lifestyle.

I believe having the tumors removed and then doing everything possible to nurture my immune system allowed my body to heal. Now that I have the knowledge of what I can do to support my body's defenses and activate its natural healing ability, I must continue to use that knowledge to live a long, healthy, active life.

In the weeks and months immediately following the completion of your treatment, you must remember to be conscious of your physical health. Getting rest is as important now as it was during your recovery process. You can't expect to do everything you did the way you did it before the cancer and not be exhausted or overwhelmed. Even though you feel as though you are "well" and your doctors agree, you are still healing. It will take time to re-establish your mental and physical stamina.

You must be aware of your mental and emotional health. Learn to take your time and stay away from toxic relationships and negative people. Be kind to yourself. Take time to enjoy life. Continue to be creative. If you took up a new hobby during your illness, continue to pursue it or find a new more exciting way to express your creativity.

Don't be afraid to ask for help. People often don't know you need help unless you ask. It is not a sign of weakness or lack of control to ask for help. It is the smart thing to do. Don't lift things that are too heavy. You shouldn't have been doing it before you were ill. Don't do it now. You are not indestructible, even if you've always made it appear that you are.

Re-evaluate your life. Are you doing what you want to do? You have no control over the quantity of life you have left to live. You do have control over HOW you will live. Make the decision now to turn the rest of your years into a quality life.

The information on the next few pages is a summary and guide that you can refer to and follow as you go through treatment, continue your healing process, and transition into a new and completely different, healthy lifestyle. Keep it handy.

Be Cautious In Decision Making

- Take your time making your decision. Don't let doctors or anyone else rush you into a decision that might not be right for you. Your treatment choice is one of the most important decisions you will ever make.

- Get more than one opinion. Don't accept the first recommended treatment plan as your only option.

- Ask questions. If you don't get answers, ask again and again until you do.

- Be informed. Read everything you can find about your type of cancer and any treatment possibilities.

- Postpone any major decision, if possible — including medical, until you have time to think.

- Keep other decision making to a minimum. Your judgment may be clouded at this time. If need be, get someone to "walk you through" your day.

- Ask family, friends, or associates whom you trust to make minor decisions for you.

- Wisdom has three components: love, firmness, and knowledge. Look for these traits in the people from whom you seek and accept guidance.

- Delegate everything you possibly can, except decisions about your treatment.

- Beware of anyone whose well-meaning advice contains such words as: "should," "you better," "it's time you," or "you must." Some people are just "busy bodies" and could be giving you the wrong advice.

Be Gentle With Yourself

- Be gentle, kind, and tender with yourself.

- Accept the fact that it may take a while before you are completely well.

- Treat yourself with the same degree of care and affection you would a good friend in a similar situation.

- Don't take on new responsibilities during this time. Let your employer and co-workers know you've suffered an illness and are healing.

- If at all possible, avoid situations in which you are stressed or upset. My sister's death was unexpected and unavoidable. I had to allow myself to feel the emotion.

- Accept assistance and support when offered, and ask for these when you need them.

- Experience any feelings of sadness, fear, and pain when they arise, but don't dwell on them. These are a natural result of a diagnosis of a life threatening disease.

- Don't be hard on yourself, if you cry. Crying has its own specialness; a cleansing, purifying release. God gave you tear ducts for one reason…to cry.

- Don't rush around. Your body needs energy for repair.

- Pray, meditate, and rest.

- Go to bed earlier and sleep a little later. Rest is the foundational building block of health.

Be With The Emotional Pain

- If you are having emotional pain, be with it. Experience it. Don't deny it, cover it, or run away from it.

- To feel emotional pain after a diagnosis of a life threatening disease is normal, natural, proof that you are alive, a sign that you are able to respond to life's experiences.

- Understand that emotional pain is a part of healing.

- Don't become "heavily involved" in anything except your well being (especially other people's drama.)

Anticipate A Positive Outcome

- Focus on a positive outcome. Whatever we focus on, expect, anticipate, plan, and act upon is what we attract.

- Decide there is nothing more important in your life right now than your goal of getting well. This will require daily discipline.

- Create a plan to become healthy again. Seek out doctors, nutritionists, and massage therapists. I call them my personal maintenance crew.

- Work in partnership with your maintenance crew. Even though I took the naturopathic route, my oncologist insists on a bimonthly blood test to read my cancer marker numbers and note any changes. This is important to the maintenance of good health.

- In the beginning, conduct a monthly review of your progress. Later on, you may be able to go to every other month or quarterly.

Give Yourself Time To Heal

- The healing process takes time.

- The further along the dis-ease, the more time and discipline it will take to heal. In this age of fast foods and instantly replaceable everything, it's hard to accept that anything takes time.

- Give yourself the luxury of time. You require enormous amounts of time for yourself now: time to rest, pray, meditate, plan your meals, be creative, be physically active and socialize with positive people.

- Guard your time. Stay away from negative people and circumstances.

- Be aware that much of your energy is being used for healing and this is your number one priority.

Nourish Your Body

- Give your body what it needs to function properly.

- Assess your current food stock and get rid of anything in your house that you shouldn't be eating. Find out what foods and supplements are right for you. Be aware of what foods you eat.

- Avoid anything that interferes with the proper functioning of your body.

- Drink lots of water…eight to ten glasses per day.

- Eat fresh fruits and vegetables. Wash them thoroughly to be sure there are no remnants of pesticides and then eat them raw or lightly steamed.

- If you insist on eating meat, eat only organic meats and other protein products which are free of hormones and chemicals often used to fatten up animals before market.

- Eat only wild fish, not farm fed. You don't want to know what is in the food the farm fed fish are eating and you certainly don't want to put it in your body.

- Reduce your intake of caffeine, nicotine, artificial sweeteners, and alcohol.

- Don't eat junk food or foods that contain sugar. Cancer feeds on sugar.

- Don't eat dairy products as they create mucus. Cancer thrives in mucus.

- Take a good multi-vitamin/mineral supplement. Especially valuable are Vitamins A, B, C, D3, and E, magnesium, and folic acid.

Maintain A Positive Attitude

- Your happiness during this time is dependent on your attitude. Happiness is a choice. Make the decision to be happy in spite of your situation.

- Take control of your situation.

- Repeat your affirmations several times a day.

- Productive work often helps emotions. Do as much of it as you feel comfortable doing.

- Don't let others convince you to do things. Do what you believe is right for you.

- Guard your emotional and mental health at all times. Don't try to understand, comprehend, or figure things out.

- Don't blame yourself for getting the "dis-ease." Forgive yourself for anything you feel you did wrong and do things differently

- Use your visualization techniques daily. Visualize yourself healthy and happy, doing the things you want to do.

- Healing is a process. You have the right to process in your own way.

Create A Living Environment

- Invite other living things into your environment such as plants, flowers, pets, goldfish, or birds. I have two incredible Burmese cats and I hung a hummingbird feeder on my back patio. Both the cats and I love to watch the birds.

- Redecorate your living space or buy some new clothes.

- Be sure your household cleansers are safe.

- Invite friends and family to come for a meal, pot luck preferred. Then, they bring the food. (Be sure they are aware ahead of time what you can and can't eat.)

- Meet your neighbors.

- Open the curtains and let the sun in.

- Open a window and enjoy the fresh air.

- Practice deep breathing. Place your hand on your heart, breast, stomach, or any part of your body that seems to be in turmoil. Breathe into that area. Tell yourself, "I am healthy and all is well."

- Don't isolate yourself from others.

Pamper Yourself

- Take time for yourself.

- Take hot, bubble baths. Create atmosphere in the bathroom. Light scented candles, play soft music.

- Get a massage. I found an incredible masseur who not only gave my body healing therapy, he helped me renew my spirit and learn to live a more peaceful, stress free life.

- Get a manicure and a pedicure.

- Get a facial.

- Have your hair done.

- Bask in the sun.

- Read a trashy novel.

- Visit a museum

- See.a play, opera, or ballet.

- Take art lessons. For me, this was better than therapy.

- Take ballroom dance lessons. This is not only exercise, it's a way to be touched in a positive manner. My dance teacher and I laughed and laughed releasing endorphins and helping me heal.

- Buy yourself something frivolous, or something you've always wanted.

- Send yourself a bouquet of flowers.

- Watch the movie, "Last Holiday," and take the trip you've always dreamed of.

- Alternate rest with activity. This will bring efficient healing.

Pay Attention To Your Sleep Patterns And Your Dreams

- Healing is a full-time process, 24 hours a day, even while you are sleeping...especially then.

- Changes in sleep patterns are common when healing. You may sleep longer or require an afternoon nap.

- Be careful what you watch on television before going to sleep. News that makes you angry and movies that create fear are not healthy and often disrupt your sleep.

- Prepare for sleep by turning off the television, taking a long, hot bath, putting on something pretty to sleep in and crawling into bed. Use battery operated flicker candles to create a soft, peaceful mood in your bedroom. These are much safer than real candles.

- You may get messages, information, insights, or lessons in your dreams. Be open to them.

- If you have problems falling asleep or staying asleep, don't worry. Do something nurturing for yourself instead. Listen to soft music, pray, meditate, or read something inspiring for a while.

- If you are awake in the wee hours, talk with God. This is a wonderful time to tell Him what you feel, ask for what you want and need, and listen for His answers.

- Keep a notebook and pen by your bed to write down any thoughts you may have or messages you receive during the night.

Make Changes

- A new chapter in your life has begun.

- Know that you have the ability to make the changes required.

- You will probably need to eat differently, exercise more, sleep more, add affirmations, visualization, meditation, and prayer to your life.

- Expect to discover a stronger, different, more evolved you.

- Don't be surprised if you find yourself to be more independent, more confident, and happier.

- Be prepared to make adjustments and modifications.

- Embrace your new life. You have survived an ordeal.

- Start experimenting with new ways of doing things.

- Let yourself enjoy the excitement of uncertainty.

Surround Yourself With Loving, Healing Light

- Ask God to surround you with loving, healing light.

- Let this light fill every cell of your body. Breathe it into all areas that need healing whether they be physical, mental, or spiritual.

- Pray, asking for the strength to endure, the power to heal, and the courage to live life abundantly.

Celebrate

- Throw an "I Kicked Cancer's Butt" party.

- Invite everyone who helped in your survival, healing, and growth.

- Acknowledge the help and support you received from others. Send thank you notes, flowers, gifts, or whatever is appropriate.

- When you come across others in need, remember, the value of the help you received.

- Give yourself a pat on the back for a job well done. Better yet, give yourself something you've been wanting for a long time.

- You've been through dis-ease, surviving, healing, growing, and becoming

- Now, it's time for celebrating!!!

A Final Note

THIS EXPERIENCE HAS TRULY BEEN A SPIRITUAL JOURNEY. THE BATTLE has been more psychological than physical. Cancer has reshaped my life. It has brought me to a new appreciation of my life, helped me discover talents I never knew I had, and taught me to make better choices in my daily life. Those choices range from the foods with which I nourish my body, to exercise, to the people I associate with, and the relationships I encourage.

I have come to a very clear understanding of what is really important in my life — what my priorities are regarding who I want to spend time with and how I want to spend the rest of my life, however long that may be. I have learned the value of "now," and I concentrate on being fully present in that now. I've learned to be more tolerant with people and a bit more compassionate. I've learned to be less judgmental and more accepting. Most of all, I've learned to be grateful for every day and each breath.

I thank my body for the lessons received during this healing journey. I have learned to:

- not let people, no matter how expert, rush me into making decisions.
- eat only the foods that will nourish my body and give me energy
- stop when I'm tired and rest

- spend time with the people I love and stay away from those who offer nothing positive to the quality of the moments of my life.

- compare the cost of treatment to the cost of poor health

- do things, go places, and be with people because it's what I want

- Most of all, I have learned to trust God 100%.

I may not fully understand why this happened to me, but I know for absolute positive sure He has guided me through it. Good things have come about because of the cancer. If I hadn't had the surgery, I wouldn't have spent time recuperating at my sister's home right before she died. I wouldn't have had the quality time with her which I cherish. I've made new friends. I've been asked by doctors and technicians at the medical offices I've visited to speak to some other patients who need someone to support them through their cancer experiences. I've lost weight and can get back into some of my beautiful suits that had gotten more than a bit snug. I see many more good things coming my way in the future.

Since my cancer adventure began, two of my friends have been diagnosed with breast cancer and have died. This is partly why I decided to write this book. Should you have such a diagnosis, take responsibility for your own health. Whether you choose to go the "holistic" route, stick with conventional treatment, or do a combination of the two, which I did, I want to encourage you to boost your immune system and create wellness in your life

Don't listen to people who tell you that you only have a year to live or that you may have five more years. Only God knows how much time you have left. No human can predict your response to your illness. They don't know how determined you are to live or what you are willing to do to create and maintain a healthy lifestyle. I chose not to focus on the negative messages given to me by many health care professionals. I have a lot to do yet in this lifetime, and I intend to get it done. God has a job for me, and I am going to do everything I can to fulfill His purpose for my life. I decided to get well and live.

It reminds me of that poem by Robert Frost which says, "*...two roads diverged and I...I chose the one less travelled by.*" Well, our two roads are either the road of passivity and despair or the road of action and hope. I chose the latter. I felt God and I together could make me well and whole again, if only I stayed focused on the possibilities.

We make choices every moment of every day. When we choose to trust God, take part in creating our own destiny, show gratitude for the progress we've already made and stay focused forward, we will see miracles at every turn. Then and only then are we moving toward a future filled with unlimited possibilities. Faith is the confident assurance that something we believe is true or something we desire is going to happen.

Affirm each day that you are well. Say to yourself each morning, "I believe God has a purpose for my life and I intend to live a long, healthy life to fulfill that purpose." Then take the action required to make that happen. Keep your thoughts positive, make better choices, and remember, "The Power that made the body, heals the body. There is no other way."

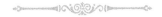

Supporting A Cancer Patient

Supporting A Cancer Patient

CANCER OR ANY MAJOR ILLNESS IS HARD ON THE FAMILY, FRIENDS, and caretakers as well as the patient. No one likes to be confronted with a situation that stirs up terrible fears and hurt, but there are priceless lessons we can learn while enduring them. If you are supporting someone who is going through a health trial, there are many things to consider and remember. A crucial element is that you must take care of you. You can't take care of anyone else if you are tired, worn out, or sick.

Before you offer help, consider:

- Diagnosis of serious illness changes people — even before their treatment begins

- Commitment to being an ongoing friend throughout the entire cancer process may be a long and tedious time.

- Your job will be to help her discover what she needs, and be there to support her, not to express your opinions about her situation.

- Discussion with the person about the disease should only be done if you are comfortable talking about it. If you are not comfortable or you don't have an open mind, keep your opinions to yourself.

- It is important for you to learn all you can about the disease. (Both the internet and your local library have an abundance of information about most major illnesses.)

- You absolutely must stay positive no matter how negative the ill person becomes.

- You need to accept her feelings. Don't try to talk her out of them. She feels what she feels and if she can't express those freely, without judgment from you, she may clam up and become withdrawn.

- She may not be able to express her emotions easily. If that's the case, don't try to force her to talk about them.

- She may express anger at God. You don't need to defend God. He's got the big picture. He understands.

- The ill person may not handle this situation the way you would. She will respond in the way most natural to her personality. Accept that different people handle problems in different ways.

- This experience can be an opportunity to learn more about yourself.

Once you've accepted the challenge, things to do include:

- Let her talk as much or as little about her diagnosis and prognosis as she chooses.

- Be slow to offer advice, even if she asks you.

- Let the seriousness of the disease determine the amount of time and commitment you offer.

- Help the person find as many ways as possible to face the new phase in her life.

- Pray for the person every day.

- Before you pray, ask the person if she would like you to pray for healing, peace, God's will, or if she has some other prayer request. Respect her wishes.

- Pray with her. If appropriate, hold her hand or touch her shoulder. The human touch is powerful, and it makes a human connection. Be careful not to make her uncomfortable by touching too much or hugging too long. I have one friend who consistently hugged me just a bit too long for my liking. It sometimes made me wonder if she thought I was moving on to the next world right then.

- If the person is in pain, keep the visit short.

- Sit silently with the person sometimes. Or bring a book and read, but be there with her.

- Allow the person to cry. Crying is a step toward healing.

- If you feel like crying, cry.

- Offer to drive the person for any kind of medical treatments she may be undergoing i.e. chemotherapy, radiation treatments or natural vitamin infusions.

- Offer to do practical things, such as clean the house, do the laundry or shopping, assist in answering letters and cards, mow the lawn, or make phone calls.

- Encourage the person to join a support group for survivors of her type of illness.

- Be willing to listen to her worries and concerns, especially, "Will my cancer recur?" "What will happen if I die?" You don't have to provide an answer, just listen.

- Think about tangible things you can do that say, "I care." One friend's wife brought me six quarts of various homemade soups. That was greatly appreciated. A young woman from my church, who lives in the same town and had previously experienced cancer herself, wrote me a weekly chatty letter telling me what she was doing in her life, how her kids were, and the positive things she was observing in the world. I looked forward to receiving her notes because she was so upbeat and it took my mind off my experience.

- Plan celebrations for every anniversary of being cancer free.

- Plan a big party when the person passes the five-year mark.

- If the person with cancer knows it's terminal, help to plan a family reunion. Make it a time when people can lovingly say goodbye. Ask those who can't attend the event to write a letter to express their love.

- Arrange for a family picture with as many relatives and close friends as possible.

Whatever you do:

- Don't ask, "How are you?" Instead, ask, "Do you feel like talking?"

- Don't be afraid of the word "cancer" or "tumor." If you're afraid to use such words, the person may sense your discomfort and hold back.

- Don't say "Let me know if you need anything." I had a friend who did this to me. "I'm here. Call me if you need me. I don't want to bother you." I know she meant well, but I didn't even know what I needed other than friendship. It would have meant so much to have her call occasionally and just say, "I was thinking of you."

- Don't say, "I know how you feel." You don't KNOW how anyone else feels. You can only guess.

- Don't say things like, "This was God's will. You must be strong. You should count your blessings that it's not worse."

- Don't ask things like "What did you do to bring this on yourself?"

- Don't be afraid to discuss the progress of the disease.

- Don't give false hope, but don't discourage.

- Don't treat her as an invalid unless she is an invalid.

- Don't try to comfort her by describing how badly you or someone else suffered during surgery, radiation, or chemotherapy.

- Don't tell horror stories. (My sister-in-law had the same thing as you and after suffering terribly for a year, she died.)

- If you feel she is unrealistically optimistic, don't attempt to convince her of your reality.

- Don't push the person to try alternative medicine or find another doctor. If she asks for that kind of help, offer to do research or refer her to someone who can assist her.

- Don't talk to her about living wills, a legal power of attorney, and a medical power of attorney, unless you are the appropriate person.

- Don't take it upon yourself to feng shui her house, get rid of any of her things, or repot her plants. I promise you, it's not appreciated.

About The Author

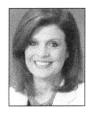 JUDI MOREO HAS HAD AN INCREDIBLE LIFE. SHE HAS been a journalist, a secretary, a model, a finishing school and model agency owner, a professional speaker, an award-winning author, a corporate executive, an entrepreneur, a consultant, and a cancer survivor.

She has always believed that "life is an adventure" and her adventurous nature has taken her to twenty-eight countries around the world. But all of her adventures have not been glamorous. Judi works, struggles, and perseveres. She is a real woman whose life isn't sprinkled with pixie dust. She has learned to make things happen for herself, and she has shared much of that knowledge with you in this book. These are valuable lessons acquired throughout her life and on her journey through cancer.

Around the globe, there are many women (and men) whose lives are a testimony to Judi's personal and professional success. She is a prolific writer and an amazing public speaker, her programs and training sessions provide positive opportunities for more complete inner knowledge and personal fulfillment.

It is no wonder that she has a collection of awards, but to her "life is not about the awards. It is about the reward of making a difference in another person's life." And that, she has done over and over and over again.

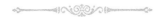

Appendix

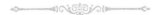

Charlotte's Oatmeal Cookies

3	Ripe Bananas
2 c.	Rolled Oats (Old fashioned/not Quick)
1 c.	Dates (pitted and chopped,) or cherries, dried apricots, dried cranberries, raisins or a combination of these
1/2 c.	Walnuts or pecans
1/3 c	Vegetable or flax oil
1 t.	Vanilla extract

Preparation:

Preheat oven to 350 degrees F (175 degrees C)

In a large bowl, mash the bananas. Stir in oats, fruit, nuts, oil and vanilla. Mix well. Allow to stand for 15 minutes. Drop by teaspoonful onto an ungreased cookie sheet.

Bake for 20 minutes in the preheated oven until lightly brown.

Note: The riper the banana, the sweeter the cookie. You can also use a bit of Agave Nectar to make a sweeter cookie, but be sure to reduce the amount of oil you use. We have sometimes added flax seed and sesame seed for a crunchier cookie.

Essiac Tea

Supplies Needed
Do not use anything made of aluminum.

Stainless steel kettle with lid (or glass)

Stainless steel sieve

Large stainless steel or wood stirring utensil

Stainless steel funnel or 2-cup glass measuring cup

Glass bottles can be colored or clear glass

3 gallon kettle and 14 bottles are ideal for 1 cup herb mix + 2 gallons of water.

Sterilize bottles and lids

To make 1 cup of mix to brew with 2 gallons of distilled water:

Burdock root (cut)	=	1/2 cup
Sheep Sorrel (powdered)	=	3/8 cup
Slippery Elm bark (powdered)	=	2 Tablespoons + 2 teaspoons
Turkey rhubarb (powdered)	=	1 teaspoon

The water you use for making Essiac tea should be as pure as possible. Don't use tap water. Most people use distilled water.

1. Mix dry ingredients thoroughly.

2. Measure out desired amount of dry ingredients.

3. Pour water into pot.

4. Bring water to a rolling boil with the lid on.

continued next page

5. Stir dry ingredients into boiling water.

6. Replace lid and continue boiling at reduced heat for 10 minutes.

7. Turn off fire. Scrape down sides of pot and stir mixture thoroughly.

8. Replace lid, let pot sit and cool undisturbed for 10-12 hours (overnight).

9. Reheat to steaming hot, but do not boil.

10. Turn off heat and allow herbs to settle for a few minutes.

11. Pour hot liquid through sieve to catch sediment.

12. Use funnel to fill sterilized bottles, put lids on.

13. Allow bottles to cool, then tighten lids.

14. Store in dark cool place.

15. Always refrigerate any opened bottle.

16. Discard, if mold develops.

17. Unopened bottles can be stored in a cool, dark place, or keep all the bottles in the refrigerator. Don't freeze Essiac or warm it up in a microwave. If you need to dilute it, just add hot water.

Directions for Use

Drink 1 fluid ounce Essiac tea per day, diluted in 2 fluid ounces hot water. This should be sipped, preferably at bedtime on an empty stomach. Food should not be eaten within one hour before or after drinking the tea.

Dry Brushing

Use a complexion brush and brush the entire body once a day, preferably first thing in the morning. It should take about 15 minutes to give yourself a thorough skin brushing. Always dry brush your dry and naked body before you shower or bathe because you will want to wash off the impurities from the skin which result from the brushing action.

You can do the brushing from your head-to-toe or toe-to-head. It really doesn't matter as long as you brush toward the heart, not away from it. Use long, sweeping strokes starting from the bottom of your feet upwards, from your hands toward your shoulders, and on the torso, in an upward direction to assist the lymph circulation back to your heart. Use circular counter clockwise strokes on the abdomen. Use light pressure, except on areas where the skin is thick such as the soles of your feet. Especially use very light pressure on the breasts. Brush upwards on your back and down from the neck. Better yet, have someone else brush your back. Be sure to remind them to use light pressure.

After getting out of the shower, dry off vigorously and massage your skin with pure plant oils such as avocado, apricot, almond, olive, or sesame.

Cleanse your brush using soap and water a minimum of once a week, rinse well, and dry in an open, sunny spot to prevent mildew.

Meditation

Simply relax with your eyes closed. Pay attention to your breathing. See if you can slow your breathing down as if you are sleeping. Feel the air come in through your nose each time you inhale. Imagine that air is caressing your face and your soul. Feel your breath leave as you exhale. Each time you exhale, imagine tension is leaving your body.

Then as you breathe in, imagine the air going up your nose is spreading relaxation up into the top of your head. As you exhale, imagine the tension leaving your head and your body. Continue to breathe in and out, expanding the areas of your body that you cleanse with your breathe. Focus on one part of your body at a time until you have thought about your entire body and the tension leaving each part.

This process will take a few minutes. You can do it as slowly or as quickly as you like. When you finish, sit quietly for two or three minutes.

Other Life Affirming Products from Judi Moreo

You Are More Than Enough: Every Woman's Guide to Purpose, Passion & Power

You Are More Than Enough is a powerful guide to discovering your purpose, unleashing your passion and shaping your habits to realize the success you want in all the areas of your life — personal and professional relationships, career, finances, and security. In this book, Judi translates her wealth of knowledge and practical experience into a meaningful and motivating guide. Writing in a comfortable, conversational style, she gives you simple, usable techniques which you can apply to your everyday world. It's like having afternoon tea with your best friend.

The moment you start to apply what you read in this book, you'll come to the realization that you really are…more than enough.

JMB1 *You Are More Than Enough* — hardback book $ 24.95
JMBJ *You Are More Than Enough* book & *Achievement Journal* $ 50.00
JMBD1 Audio Book Set — 12 CDs and *Achievement Journal* $ 99.00
JMBD2 Audio Book, Book and *Achievement Journal* $119.00

You Are More Than Enough Achievement Journal

The companion to *You Are More Than Enough*, the *Achievement Journal* is a life changing tool for setting and achieving goals. It is a method for organizing goals, dreams and expectations — as well as evaluating what's working, what's missing, and what's needed to bring positive results into your life. The *Achievement Journal* is a place to record and remind yourself of your accomplishments, successes, miracles and achievements and will keep you following your star.

JMB2 *You Are More Than Enough Achievement Journal* $34.95

continued next page

Attitude Is A Choice CD

Attitude Is A Choice offers you basic insights to help you choose the right attitude to overcome life's difficulties, build positive relationships, and discover new opportunities. When you practice Judi's ten steps of choosing the right attitude you will experience an incredible difference in your life.

JM11 *Attitude Is A Choice — CD* $19.95

Communication Is A Choice CD

Communication Is A Choice offers you easy communication techniques to help you say the right thing at the right time in order to connect with others in an effective and persuasive style. Communication is the number one problem in relationships today...whether they be professional or personal. Don't let it be a problem for you!

JM17 *Communication Is A Choice CD* $19.95

Life Choices

The *Life Choices* books are a series in which real people share their stories of overcoming obstacles, putting lives back together and following their passions to create successful, significant lives.

While the stories shared differ in context, they share a common thread of courage, hope and fulfillment. No matter what obstacles you encounter, or how many pieces your life is in, there is a way to find a new path, make a new choice and create a better life.

In the pages of these books, you will discover how the authors have taken a variety of paths to find their own way back to wholeness and success. They may be the inspiration for you to continue your journey, make new choices and create a new life.

LC1 *Life Choices: Navigating Difficult Paths*	$24.95
LC2 *Life Choices: Putting The Pieces Together*	$24.95
LC3 *Life Choices: Pursuing Your Passion*	$24.95
LC4 *Life Choices: It's Never Too Late*	$24.95
LC5 *Life Choices: Ways to Wellness*	$24.95

Overcoming Cancer

If you would like to order multiple copies of *Overcoming Cancer, A Journey of Faith*, please call 702-896-2228. Discounts are available on quantity orders.

Speaking Engagements

Judi Moreo is available for speaking engagements. If you would like to have her make a presentation for your organization, you may contact Turning Point International at (702) 896-2228 or contact Judi directly via e-mail at judi@judimoreo.com . For more information about Judi, visit her website www.judimoreo.com.

Continuing Inspiration

If you would like to receive Judi's monthly newsletter "Winning Solutions," sign up at www.judimoreo.com.

To read more of Judi's journey and for continuing support and inspiration, please visit www.cancerwakeupcall.com.

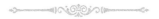

Order by phone: (702) 896-2228

Order online: www.judimoreo.com or www.lifechoicesbook.com

Recommended Reading

In addition to the many essays and articles I read on line, the following is a list of some of the books I read and DVDs I watched throughout my journey.

Books

Somers, Suzanne *Knockout, Interviews With Doctors Who Are Curing Cancer and How to Prevent Getting It In The First Place,* Crown Publishers 2009

Brown, Sylvia *Psychic Healing, Using the Tools of a Medium to Cure Whatever Ails You,* Hay House 2009

Servan-Schreiber, MD, PhD, David, *Anti Cancer, A New Way Of Life,* Viking Penguin 2009

Lee, MD, John R., *What Your Doctor May Not Tell You About Breast Cancer, How Hormone Balance Can Save Your Life,* Hacette Book Group, 2003

Chopra, MD, Deepak, *Grow Younger, Live Longer, 10 Steps to Reverse Aging,* Harmony Books, 2001

Campbell, T. Colin and Campbell II, Thomas M, *The China Study, Startling Implications for Diet, Weight Loss and Long-term Health,* BenBella Books Paperback Edition, 2006

Yance Jr., Donald R, CN, MH AHG, *Herbal Medicine, Healing & Cancer, A Comprehensive Program for Prevention and Treatment.* Keats Publishing, 1999

Brazier, Brendan, *Thrive, The Vegan Nutrition Guide to Optimal Performance in Sports and Life,* DeCapo Press, 2007

Keville, Kathi *Herbs for Health and Healing, A Drug-Free Guide to Prevention and Cure,* Rodale Press, Inc., 1996

Addington, Jack Ensign, *The Secret of Healing,* Science of Mind Publications 1999

FC&A Editors, *Inner Cleansing Cures,* FC&A Publishing, 1999

Castleman, Michael, *The Healing Herbs, The Ultimate Guide to the Curative Power of Nature's Medicines,* Bantam Books 1995

Jahnke, Roger, *The Healer Within, Using Traditional Chinese Techniques to Release Your Body's Own Medicine,* Harper San Francisco,1997

Myss, Caroline, PhD, *Why People Don't Heal and How They Can,* Harmony Books 1997

DVD's
Naparstek, Belleruth, *A Meditation To Help You Fight Cancer,* Health Journeys 1991

Hay, Louise, *You Can Heal Your Life,* Hay House

Cinema Libre Distribution, Krochel Films, *Healing Cancer From The Inside Out*

Lightning Source UK Ltd.
Milton Keynes UK
UKHW022016261020
372256UK00007B/1343